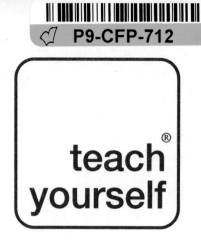

teach yourself®

pilates

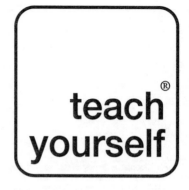

pilates
matthew aldrich

For UK order enquiries: please contact Bookpoint Ltd, 130 Milton Park, Abingdon, Oxon OX14 4SB. Telephone: +44 (0) 1235 827720. Fax: +44 (0) 1235 400454. Lines are open 09.00–18.00, Monday to Saturday, with a 24-hour message answering service. Details about our titles and how to order are available at www.teachyourself.co.uk

For USA order enquiries: please contact McGraw-Hill Customer Services, PO Box 545, Blacklick, OH 43004-0545, USA. Telephone: 1-800-722-4726. Fax: 1-614-755-5645.

For Canada order enquiries: please contact McGraw-Hill Ryerson Ltd, 300 Water St, Whitby, Ontario L1N 9B6, Canada. Telephone: 905 430 5000. Fax: 905 430 5020.

Long renowned as the authoritative source for self-guided learning – with more than 30 million copies sold worldwide – the *Teach Yourself* series includes over 300 titles in the fields of languages, crafts, hobbies, business, computing and education.

British Library Cataloguing in Publication Data: a catalogue record for this title is available from The British Library.

Library of Congress Catalog Card Number: on file.

First published in UK 2004 by Hodder Headline Ltd, 338 Euston Road, London NW1 3BH.

First published in US 2004 by Contemporary Books, a division of the McGraw Hill Companies, 1 Prudential Plaza, 130 East Randolph Street, Chicago, Illinois 60601 USA.

This edition published 2004.

The 'Teach Yourself' name is a registered trade mark of Hodder & Stoughton Ltd.

Typeset by Transet Limited, Coventry, England.
Printed in Great Britain for Hodder & Stoughton Educational, a division of Hodder Headline Ltd, 338 Euston Road, London NW1 3BH, by Cox & Wyman Ltd, Reading, Berkshire.

Papers used in this book are natural, renewable and recyclable products. They are made from wood grown in sustainable forests. The logging and manufacturing processes conform to the environmental regulations of the country of origin.

Impression number   10 9 8 7 6 5 4 3 2 1
Year   2009 2008 2007 2006 2005 2004

contents

acknowledgements

I would like to say a big thank you to everyone at Hodder who helped with this book, especially to Sue Hart who commissioned the work and to Lisa Collier for all her patient phone calls. I am very lucky to have had my forever hard-working and inspiring father behind me who, along with Averil's help, kept this book on track. To Sue: I am always in awe of the never-ending love and understanding that you show me, and that keeps me going when things get difficult. To all the people that attend my classes: this book has benefited hugely from your positive feedback. And to Taty, wherever you are in the world, I send you a big kiss and thank you for all your help with the pictures and for your encouragement.

introduction

Life is becoming more hectic as every day we are putting more demands on ourselves. In contrast to that, as a society we are becoming less physical; we spend more time sitting at a desk, in the seat of a car or slumping on sofas watching television. Suddenly we expect our bodies to jump up and do the gardening, play football, carry the kids to bed, cycle down to the park or maybe even run a marathon. We then wonder why we have to spend the rest of that week recovering before the next onslaught of activity.

There is no doubt that our bodies are designed to work in a physical way. However, the physical way we expect our bodies to move, for example the way we dig with a spade or sweep with a broom, the action of throwing or kicking a ball, the swing of a golf club or the way we carry a bag, does not always coincide with the way that our bodies should move. Many of these movements tend to be one-sided, which puts our bodies out of balance. The muscles that perform these varied tasks need to be worked regularly, and so does the infrastructure that supports them. That infrastructure is our skeleton and the muscles that surround it, especially the lower back and waist area. If our muscles are not regularly maintained and supported then they will become weak and lazy; and as our bodies become out of balance we find it more difficult to perform our daily tasks. Over a longer period of time this starts to affect the way we look, whether we are round shouldered, flat backed or slightly limping with one hip higher than the other.

Muscle imbalance is a common factor for most of us at some point in our lives, and it occurs when a particular muscle becomes too dominant or too weak for its designed range of function. This means that the muscle will either try to take over the function of another muscle group or become weaker as its partner takes control. As our bodies become physically imbalanced, this tends to affect other aspects of our lives. It can have an effect on our moods and our efficiency to carry out everyday mental and physical tasks. When this happens we put it down to not having the get-up-and-go attitude that we used to have. I put it down to not getting up and doing what we need to do!

Why Pilates?

Pilates exercises look at re-addressing the body's natural balance through focused and controlled movements. These movements aim at strengthening and lengthening your muscles with the intention of keeping your body mobile, whether just for everyday tasks or for any level of sporting activity. In Pilates we focus on the waist and lower back area. This area is the centre of support and strength for the rest of the body, giving our bodies their amazing ability to perform many and varied tasks. This must not be taken for granted, for if you do not take responsibility for maintaining your body then you cannot expect it to work well, either now or in the future.

It is a shame that most of us, and I include myself in this category, wait for something to go wrong before we fix it; we would not treat our cars that poorly.

We service our cars regularly, warm them up and even make a choice about the fuel on which they run. Think of your new Pilates programme as the regular service that you are going to give your body. Over time these exercises will make you more aware of your body shape and how you use the different muscles to support your posture through a range of movements; and once you finish your class or set of exercises the matter does not just end there. Your exercises will act as a reference point for the rest of the day about how to hold your body as you walk, sit, support your head or carry your bags. I come across many students who, even after a few classes and with an understanding of 'navel to spine' and 'drawing up', find an improvement in the strength and posture of their lower back, and they are able to gently practise these movements throughout the day without being in a class.

Pilates is not some mindless repetition of movements. It connects our mind with the way we move, so you are thinking about how you breathe and how to isolate certain movements in your body while adding stability from supporting muscle groups. This is not to say that it is a spiritual practice but more of an understanding of your body's actions and reactions to movement.

Pilates and the variations of teaching that come with it are not just a quick fix for a dodgy back, but a long-term commitment to improving posture, health and quality of life. Through regular practice, your body will feel better balanced, firmer and well poised to deal with the stresses of everyday life.

What to expect from Pilates

Pilates is suitable for almost everyone. I have worked with all age ranges – from teenagers to 90-year-olds – and they have all found it beneficial. Almost all of us tend to have a weakness somewhere in our bodies although, as a result of pain, some of us are more aware of our weaknesses than others. Locating the cause of that weakness is not always about just placing a hand on the area where it hurts and giving it a quick rub. For example, quite often back pain can be due to a muscle imbalance in one leg. Over time this can affect the way you walk, and the way you walk can compound the pain and weakness in your back. The imbalance in your body may have been building up for years before it is highlighted.

The great value of Pilates is that you can adapt your exercises to maintain your strength while improving areas of weakness. This is because you can put your body into a position of support before you begin your movements. Thus you can gently increase the intensity of your exercises as your body is strengthened and your levels of fitness increase.

Functional and structural fitness should form the basis of every fitness regime. Functional fitness means that you are training your body for what it has to do most of the time. For example, if you are a taxi or lorry driver you spend a lot of time in a cramped sitting position, possibly with a rounded back and raised shoulders. In addition there is the natural tension that goes with the job – dealing with traffic and aggressive drivers, and concentrating on where you are going. Functional fitness exercises like Pilates concentrate upon relaxing the areas of tension and strengthening the under-worked muscles. Just think for a minute if you are a professional driver with an automatic car. You are continually lifting your right leg, but have little or no movement in the left. Over time, those movements will be enough to cause an imbalance around your hip that will only compound the already weak position in your back from sitting in the car seat. Obviously, we all need to work, but with a little thought and effort we can go about our daily activities with less strain and pain in our bodies.

Without the proper support from our body, we are unable to lift ourselves safely from a chair, let alone swing a tennis racquet or golf club. Pilates should become an addition to, rather than a substitute for, any other exercise routine you might be doing. Unless you are practising at an extreme level, it does not offer a high cardiovascular workout, so to exercise your heart and to burn calories you might want to add cycling or swimming to your routine. If losing weight is your main aim then you need to look more carefully at what you are eating, as well as thinking about a balanced exercise programme.

Pilates will give you lean and long muscles, with improved posture and better co-ordination of movement around your body. Most people, when asked how they feel after an hour's Pilates class, describe sensations such as lengthened, balanced, strengthened, energized and sometimes completely 'knackered'. You get out of it what you want, and as long as you can maintain your breathing and support throughout the exercises, you choose how hard you work.

History

Joseph Pilates

Joseph Pilates was a health and fitness revolutionary. He appreciated the connection between mind and body, and was concerned with humanity's neglect of physical and mental health. Even in his day, he could see that the fast pace of living was having a disastrous effect on the strength of body and mind. He questioned many of the so-called health regimes of his time, and was always prepared to back up his belief in his fitness programmes with 'before and after' photographs showing the improvement in posture and muscle tone of his clients.

Born in Germany in 1880, Pilates as a child was frail and prone to illness. This weakness as a youngster must have inspired him to improve his fitness, for despite his fragile body he worked hard to improve his physical health. By the age of 14 he was in such good shape that he was used as a model for anatomical drawings. He studied many physical and health-related arts, including bodybuilding, boxing, diving, gymnastics and skiing. He worked in Britain as a boxer and circus performer, and even taught self-defence to English detectives.

In 1914, at the start of the First World War, Pilates was interned in Britain as a German national. This did not deter him from following his ideals and he determined to ensure the good health of his fellow prisoners by setting up exercise routines and creating exercise equipment from whatever materials he found to hand. It is said that he used the springs from the beds to create resistance exercises for the internees who were bed-ridden, so they were able to maintain some level of physical fitness that would aid their recovery. After the war he returned to Germany and by the mid-1920s he had emigrated to the USA and made his home in New York. Even though not much is known about his early years of self-study, it is evident from his writings that his knowledge was derived from many and varied health-related arts.

Pilates had an understanding of Chinese martial arts, including Kung Fu and Qi Qong. These exercises seek to promote good health through flexibility, strength, mental balance and a strong centre. Looking at his writings and exercises, it is apparent that he also had an appreciation of Indian culture and health rituals. In addition, Pilates was greatly inspired and impressed by the mental and physical attitudes adopted by early Greek civilizations. The ancient Greeks were well known for their intellect, as well as for their sporting prowess.

Such was Pilates' interest in health that he studied the movements of animals and their instinctive behaviour, which highlighted many of nature's own ways of maintaining a strong and able existence. He also noted the reactions of babies and children, and saw how muscular deformities and weaknesses could be treated and repaired at an early age.

In New York he established a Pilates studio with his wife Clara. He began working with people of varying levels of physical ability, but found a popular following in the world of dance, where his core strengthening exercises and rehabilitation movements for injuries became invaluable.

Joseph Pilates created many and varied exercises and in 1945 published his booklet, *Return to Life Through Contrology*. This set out the fundamental mat exercises that are still used today. His original mat routine was very demanding, and most of us would struggle to complete the exercises in their original form. Nevertheless most of these original exercises have been adapted to make them more usable for the varying abilities of clients who turn up to classes. Also, as new information has been discovered, so the original exercises have been enhanced, to keep them up to date.

There can be no doubt that Joseph Pilates was ahead of his time. His exercises have been around for more than 70 years, but it is only in the last ten years that their worth has been truly appreciated.

Something for the men

The few men whom I see in Pilates classes are usually there for one of two reasons: Either their physiotherapist requires it as part of some ongoing treatment or their partners have told them they must give it a go, or else. The great thing is that, when they do start coming, they soon start to realize the benefits it can have on their other physical activities. I have worked with cyclists, dancers, footballers, golfers, gymnasts, horse riders, martial arts experts and snow boarders, to name but a few. All of these sports, and many others, require and benefit from improved core strength, balance and co-ordination. Very physical sports like football and martial arts also require very balanced and precise movements to deliver the power to kick or hit properly. Where does that power come from? From our hips and waist. If Bruce Lee were alive today, I bet that he would include Pilates as an invaluable part of his exercise routine. If you look at well-trained dancers and gymnasts you will find that their exercise routines are based on many core and abdominal strengthening exercises, which is why they have such well-defined abdominal muscles. I understand that, for many men, having big biceps and shoulders makes them feel strong and possibly more attractive; but if our backs (i.e. our core muscles) are not strong enough to carry our partners across the threshold, then what's the point of big biceps?

So much for the active; what about those men who have long been inactive, perhaps by inclination or as a result of an injury? Pilates exercises can be the best starting point for gaining the fitness you have never had or for regaining that which you have lost.

The basic advice must be: Don't wait for something to break down before you decide to fix it. Most of us men appreciate that cars and machinery need to be regularly serviced, so they will keep on running and not let us down. Unfortunately it is a little more difficult to get your vertebrae or hips re-bored than it is to get new rings fitted on a piston. The core strengthening exercises in Pilates are to be added to any fitness regime you might already be practising. With additional strength in your waist and back, you will be more active for longer. My own hope is still to be surfing when I am 80!

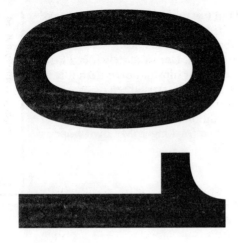

01

principles of Pilates

In this chapter you will learn:
- how to breathe correctly
- the importance of a strong centre
- the benefits of focus and fluidity.

Pilates requires a certain level of discipline in its movements and practice. Its positive effects on the body can be appreciated only by following a fundamental set of principles. Some of the movements you will be performing are subtle and slight, so these principles help to highlight that less is sometimes more. Realizing the full potential of your exercises ensures that your movements will create the strength, flexibility and improved shape we are aiming for.

Balance

In our lives we have to juggle spending time at work, time with our friends and family and also time for ourselves. For many of us it is a constant struggle not to let one area of our lives take over all our thoughts and actions. Trying to find a proper balance is not always easy, and if we fail to find it we sometimes feel unfulfilled or dissatisfied with our lot in life. The same can be said about our bodies. If we neglect one area of our body and allow another area to take over, then we do not just feel out of balance, we become out of balance. Imagine if you went to the gym and spent all your time working out on your shoulders and arms, with little or no thought for any other muscle group. Very soon you would have an impressive looking upper body, but in time you would find that the rest of your supporting structure would start to complain, as your back, knees and hips had not been strengthened to deal with the extra weight and muscle they then had to support.

Let's look at this another way: If you spend most of your day sitting down in a chair, then your knees are bent and your hips are flexed. Over time this will cause your hip flexors to become tight and your hamstrings to stiffen up. These muscles have a great effect on your posture and the shape and support of your back. Without balancing out these particular muscle groups by using stretching and strengthening exercises, the weakness will become worse. Add in the results of stooping over your desk all day, resting on your shoulders, and you will soon start to find other areas of your body suffering from lack of strength or flexibility.

A client came to me complaining of a weakness and pain down the left side of her lower back and around her hip. She was regularly seeing a physiotherapist, but the pain would return only a few days after her treatments. What was so amazing was that, physically, she had the body of a top heptathlete and the flexibility of a dancer. She trained regularly and seemed to be very knowledgeable about and very aware of her body; she knew when to rest and when to push herself. She started attending Pilates classes regularly and was soon applying the idea of core strength and support to her other movements. She said that her back felt stronger but still, by the end of the week, the pain was starting to creep back in, so we discussed potential problems that might be aggravating her situation and more specific exercises to balance out her body.

At work she spent approximately five hours at her desk and the other three hours around the office in various meetings. On talking about how she sat and moved at her desk, it turned out that she was performing over 100 side bends with an unsupported and over-extended back all on one side. By changing the set-up of her desk and moving some files and drawers around, we balanced out her movements at her work station, and after adding in a little thought about the support and shape of her back, the weakness down her left side went away. Because she was so fit, she had got away with it for many years before the weakness had become more obvious. She still attends classes and has found that, since doing Pilates, her strength and stamina in all her sports has improved.

Using a core-strengthening exercise like Pilates to balance out your body will add an invaluable support to your structure, but the idea of balance should not stop at your exercises. Once you have learned more about the exercises in this book and have a better understanding about the principles of your movements, apply these supporting principles to your body throughout the day. As far as the principle of balance goes, you can look at something as simple as carrying your shopping as part of your exercises. Keep your back supported and lengthened, your shoulder blades sliding down your back and above your hips, and transfer your weight through your pelvis into your legs while keeping your head upright. Don't forget to put an equal amount of weight in each bag, to balance out the shopping carried in each hand. Looking at other everyday tasks in the same way, if you carry a bag on one shoulder, try to alternate the shoulder you use, to balance out your movements. If you are a tradesman or a labourer, alternate which foot is forward when you are digging or bending down on one knee, and definitely think about keeping support throughout your back. When lifting your child, bend your knees and not your back; and if you carry your baby on one hip, do not always use the same hip.

Enjoying the many different oportunities life has to offer is one of the great plus points of being alive. With improved health and energy we are able to spend more time enjoying our work, socializing, holidays, days at the beach and time with loved ones; but moderation and knowing your limits is the key. We all know when we have over-indulged or overdone it, and it is important to listen to our energy levels. There seem to be some people out there who have such a strong constitution that they can exercise all day and party all night as if they have an extra-strength battery inside them. However, it will always catch up with them at some point. If you continue to overdo it, your body will soon let you know that it's time to stop, as your immune system weakens and you become ill or pick up an injury. Many top athletes, who may train up to five hours a day, often require a very strict diet and up to 14 hours' sleep a night to maintain their health and level of fitness. Listen to your body and work within your limits to find your healthy balance.

We should all accept responsibility for our actions and acknowledge the risks that we take in our activities. Most people who play racquet sports regularly will at some point have a problem with their shoulder. Regular golf players who do not make the effort to learn some body balancing and core strengthening exercises often come across some back or hip problems. Remember that most of the sports we play tend to be one-sided and do not help with the fragile balance of our bodies. Using exercises to balance out the structure of our bodies will no doubt add a more supportive quality to our physical well being. Also there is no doubt that, if we feel physically balanced, this can only help to enhance our mental balance.

Breathing

The purpose of breathing is the entry and exit of air in the lungs to supply the body with oxygen, to burn foodstuffs in the tissues and to expel waste carbon dioxide. When the body is under exertion, it requires higher levels of oxygen. Therefore, by using the various muscles in the torso, you can increase your lung capacity and your heart rate to speed up the transference of oxygen into your blood system.

To get us thinking about our breathing, we are going to look at a couple of simple breathing exercises and note how breathing can affect the shape of our body and make a difference to the way we feel. Lie down on the floor on your back, with your legs out straight, and place one hand on your chest and the other on top of your stomach. Let your feet fall sideways, relax your stomach muscles and slightly tuck in your chin to lengthen the back of your neck. Close your eyes so you will be less distracted. Breathe in gently through the nose and out through the mouth, gently drawing the air down into your lungs. Imagine that you are filling your belly with air, and feel your lower hand rise as you draw the air into the lower part of your lungs. Still on the same breath, carry on filling your lungs and feel your hand rise on your chest. Then slowly let the air escape from your lips, slightly contract your stomach muscles and let your hand sink on your belly, and relax your chest to expel the air completely from your lungs.

Try to imagine that you are filling up a balloon with water from the tap and when it is full you are squeezing the water out, starting from the bottom of the balloon, until it is empty. Keeping your breathing slow and controlled, count up to 20 breaths in and out. I hope that you have not fallen asleep but that you found this exercise quite relaxing. Breathing like this highlights the number of muscles we can use to breathe, and just like any other muscles in the body, if we do not regularly work these muscles they will become weak and inefficient.

The way we hold ourselves in our posture can greatly affect our breathing, and if this is poor over a long period of time it can be detrimental to our health. Stand up, drop your head and round your shoulders; let your stomach muscles hang out and your chest collapse. Now imagine you had to breathe in this position for the rest of your life! Of course you would not want to, but over time postural weaknesses can creep in and affect the way we breathe.

When you are breathing, the movements in the body can be abdominal, thoracic or both. In abdominal breathing, as we inhale the diaphragm is drawn down and presses on the abdominal organs, causing the abdominal wall to protrude. This increases the chest cavity, and air is drawn down into the lungs. On exhalation, the diaphragm relaxes and recoils, forcing the air out of the lungs. In thoracic breathing, the ribs are lifted by the intercostal muscles assisted by the trapezius and rhomboid muscles in the back. This increases the diameter of the chest, drawing air into the lungs; as these muscles relax, air is forced out.

For our Pilates exercises we need to pull in our stomach muscles and use thoracic breathing. To practise this, lie down on your back and place the heels of your palms onto your ribs, so that your middle fingers are touching just beneath your breast bone. Gently pull in your stomach muscles and keep your tummy flat, so that you will have to breathe out into the sides of your chest. As you breathe in, push your ribs into the palms of your hands, making your middle fingers slightly separate. As you breathe out, let your ribs come in and bring your middle fingers back together. Remember that you are not pushing your chest up; you are expanding your chest out to the sides. Practise this until you feel confident you can do it without your hands being there.

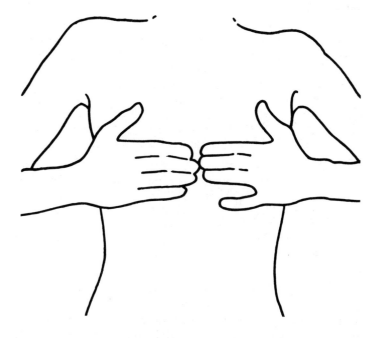

We need to maintain this thoracic breathing throughout our exercises and you will find that, as the level of exercises becomes more intense, the need for correct breathing becomes more necessary. Our aim is to build stamina into the muscles that we are working, so we must keep breathing throughout our movements. At all costs, do not hold your breath. Many of the exercises have been given a breathing pattern to help you focus on the movements and to make it easier to maintain your breathing, especially as the exercise becomes more difficult. Most people find that maintaining their breathing is the last part of the exercise to fall into place. This is normally because of having to concentrate so hard on the movements and focusing on maintaining the supporting muscles in the waist; so keep breathing, and if you find that you are holding your breath, then lower the level of intensity of your exercise.

Centring

Your abdominal muscles are part of the support structure for your spine. With strength in the centre of our bodies we are able to support and control ourselves throughout the day. Our abdominal muscles hold our internal organs in place, as well as our lower vertebrae, and without strength in this area we run the risk of prolapsed discs and organs, and compressed vertebrae and nerves. The superficial muscles of the abdomen – the rectus, transversus, internal and external obliques – help to give our centre its stability. Sitting beneath these muscles, like the bottom of a bucket, is the connective tissue of the pelvic floor.

Whenever balancing, lifting, running, throwing or walking we rely on these muscles for control, support and strength. When there is a weakness in our abdominal muscles, the situation is similar to that of a 20-storey building with the two middle floors made of rubber; the top floors have no proper support and cannot maintain their stability. To test this theory stand up and balance on one leg. Now carefully start to lift the heel of the foot on which you are standing. As you come up onto the ball of your foot, you will start to notice yourself getting wobbly; as you go higher your shoulders will start to move more to compensate for your imbalance. Set your foot down and do the same exercise again, but this time draw your navel towards your spine as you pull your stomach muscles in. You will notice that there is less movement in your shoulders and it is easier to balance. If we add some focus into this exercise by looking at a fixed point on the wall, this will improve your balance and make you feel more centred on the spot. Working and moving our bodies with a supported centre gives us more balance and control. Pilates exercises remind us how to use and strengthen our important core muscles, and also show our bodies how to work from a supported centre.

If you have ever watched 'the world's strongest man' on television or seen weight lifters in a gym, you will often have seen them tightly strapping on a thick belt to support their back before they lift a heavy weight. I would not want to be the one to tell them, but if they had spent more time strengthening their back and abdominal muscles, they would not need a supporting belt. Your natural belt is the band of muscles that run around your waist, so you do not need the support of a belt if you strengthen and engage these muscles.

Many techniques and arts look at moving the body from a strong centre. Martial arts such as Karate, Kung Fu and Tai Chi rely on building up the energy within the centre. All good dancers rely on a strong waist to support their elegant movements and to give them control over their balance. In Yoga, if you engage your moolabandha, you draw up your pelvic floor and abdominal muscles to support your spine and internal organs. With the Alexander Technique, you learn how to put your body into a position of support for your back before you move.

Starting your exercises with a strong centre means that you are supporting the position of your back throughout your movements. In our exercises we may be using anything from 25 up to 80 per cent of the strength in our abdominal muscles, depending on the level we want to achieve. Over time, as you get used to engaging the muscles in your centre, it will become second nature to support your waist before moving your body.

Control and isolation

Try this exercise and do not worry if you have a difficult time trying to accomplish it: Stand up straight on your bare feet and wiggle all your toes to loosen up your feet. Now keep your big toe pushed into the floor while you lift the other four toes off the floor. If you do not find this too difficult, then replace each of those four toes back on the floor, one at a time, while still pushing your big toe into the floor. If you can do that, then try keeping your four smaller toes on the floor while you lift and lower the big toe away from the floor and back down. For almost all of us, this is going to be a difficult exercise, because how often do we need to use our toes individually? Most of the time, if we walk anywhere, we are wearing shoes and walking on a flat surface. Remember that our feet were originally designed to walk over uneven surfaces and to grip with our toes when balancing or climbing. Take a look at chimpanzees and you will see that they have as much control with their feet as we do with our hands. Obviously we have evolved a little since then, and we have not so much need for this level of control, but if you were recovering from a damaged ankle or foot, you might need to perform such exercises to regain control of particular muscles in your foot, in order to maintain the balance of muscle use when you walk.

Going back to that exercise, let's see if we can make it a little easier by isolating the movement with some help from our hands. Put your finger on your big toe and gently hold it in place as you lift your other toes off the floor. Add the same idea to the rest of the exercises by isolating the area you want to keep fixed, and move the other toes. You will then find it easier to perform the movements, and if you carried on practising, in time you would be able to move each toe individually. As you add this idea of isolating one area, it makes it easier to target a specific area of movement. This means that you can focus on building strength into possible areas of weakness, which are often neglected.

A common exercise that many men perform in gyms is the bicep curl. In this exercise it is very tempting to try lifting too much weight at the expense of good form and supported movement. Ideally, in this exercise you keep your back fixed and your shoulder blades down as you lift the weight towards you and lower it with control. If the weight is too heavy, then you start to feel more movement in your back and shoulders to get the weight up and down. This is fine if you want to exercise your back and shoulders, and you are completely aware of engaging all those muscles in those areas and you are working from a position of support, but this is a potentially damaging exercise for your back if you are not! Your shoulders and arms may be strong enough to lift the weight, but without proper training your back can lack the strength to support you through this movement. To build up strength, taking a lighter weight and engaging your abdominal muscles while keeping your spine fixed would be a much better way of performing this exercise.

Adding a level of control to our movements, and thinking before we move, can give us more confidence in our everyday actions – whether we are gardening, bent over fixing the car or carrying children. Having more control through our exercises lets us appreciate the varying muscles in our bodies and how they work. Through regular practice muscle memory will improve, and as the control of movement and awareness in your actions gets better, it will again become second nature for you to engage the muscles in your centre before you carry, lift, throw, hit or get up off the floor. You owe it to your body to give it a decent level of control, as without this your body will never reach its physical potential, whatever your age. You can decide for yourself whether having increased control over your physical abilities will add to an improvement in your mental well being. For me, clarity of movement is the basis for a healthy body and a healthier mind.

Focus

How often do our minds wander and jump from decision to indecision, or our thoughts get caught up in an almost endless circle with no definite answers? With so many choices and distractions in life, it is sometimes difficult to focus. We need to work out what is important in our lives, and get on with enjoying it, rather than worrying about what we do not have and probably do not need. We definitely need our bodies to work with us rather than against us. With focus on our movements and our actions, we can isolate the exact areas in our bodies that need strengthening.

With many of the exercises you will perform, you are trying to pinpoint the exact movement of particular muscle groups, while holding other parts of your body in isolation and controlling your breathing. By focusing on every movement, we can soon improve our muscle memory and make the exercises more exact and beneficial. With this clarity in our movement, we can start to appreciate the knock-on effect of our every action and begin to achieve a better balance in our bodies.

Think about this: When you walk up the stairs, how many different muscles do you use? Try it for yourself. Stand up and lift your right leg off the floor with your knee bent, without leaning back, and keep your shoulders level. What are the first muscles that you start to notice? Probably the muscles in your thigh, then the muscles in your left foot as they continually adjust to keep your balance. Now think about all the other muscles that you need to support this more balanced position so you do not fall over. The muscles in your waist are trying to keep your pelvis level; the muscles in your torso are engaging to stop you leaning over to one side, and even the muscles around your neck and shoulders are working harder to keep you upright. All this to take one step!

Focus on movements can be learned. Over time, as you keep performing your exercises, your actions will become more fluid and efficient, and your level of concentration will improve. This will no doubt have a knock-on effect, not only in your physical actions but also in your mental clarity. If you have ever watched people practising Tai Chi or Yoga, you will have noticed that they are focusing on their breathing, balance, posture and exact movement and direction. In these movements there is no time to waste in having thoughts elsewhere. By adding focus to your exercises, you really can target the areas of possible imbalance, enabling you to appreciate your own weaknesses and strengths, and therefore placing yourself in the best position to get your body into better shape. As you start to become more aware of how your body moves, you will learn to support yourself throughout the day.

I wonder how many of us have been taught how to pick things up correctly? If you are in a job where you are continually lifting light or heavy objects, then at some point someone should have explained to you the safe practice of carrying and lifting. If you are picking up a heavy box then you should keep your back in a lengthened position, bend your knees and keep your shoulder blades down, so that you are using the big muscles in your legs and keeping your back in a supported position. Ideally, you should engage the muscles in your waist before you lift, so that they can maintain the support in your back. In reality, how many of us, with little or no thought about our backs, bend over to pick up many different objects, until one day the twinge occurs that turns into a never-ending on and off muscle ache? By focusing on your movements throughout your exercises, you will be reminding your body of all the necessary muscles that you need to perform the simplest of tasks. With just a little more concentration on our movements, we can work with our bodies to get more out of them and add hours of efficiency to our day.

Fluidity

Except when resting or eating, our bodies are designed to be on the move; indeed, many of us find great discomfort in sitting still for too long. If you look at children, it is difficult to get them to sit still for long – and understandably so. As children we run around, building up our strength and movement skills for later life. Unfortunately, no one warns children that their later life may be spent sitting down even more than they did at school. Remember that our bodies are not designed to sit in chairs, and most chairs are not designed for our bodies. I am sure that, when Neanderthal man had the choice of sitting on a flat rock or squatting, he chose to squat. We should spend more time thinking about what is good for our bodies, rather than what we think looks good for them.

As adults many of us crave movement, and we find it through sport, dance or outdoor activities – anything from golf to whitewater rafting. Many injuries occur when there is a sudden jolt or an over-extending movement within our bodies. If you can train your body to be more aware of your range of movement, and to support your joints, then the chances of injury are greatly reduced. If you regularly play sport then you should think about adding support exercises into your training; if you spend most of the time sitting down then you must train your body to deal with the effects that sitting has on your body.

With your Pilates exercises you are trying to make your movements seamless and smooth. Think of your body as strong elastic, and as you reach the limit of a movement, gently recoil and return, keeping a continuous flow throughout. Some of the movements can be performed with more speed, but never jerkily or erratically. Slowing down our movements can often be a way of adding intensity and support into many exercises.

If you are not already on the floor then sit down and do a couple of sit-ups. Now do the same sit-up, but pull in your stomach muscles and take 20 seconds to come up to a sitting position, and another 20 seconds to roll yourself back onto the floor. Keep a smooth and controlled movement throughout, and at no point stop or jerk yourself forward or back. It makes it more difficult, doesn't it? However, with that sense of gradual movement you can really feel which muscles are working and how the rest of your body reacts to the exercise. If you do the exercise quickly, you just throw your head and shoulders forward to get yourself up. Do not worry if you could not actually get all the way up! By the end of this book, you will be able to do it.

Adding this idea of fluid movement into your exercises helps you to listen to and be more aware of how your body moves and its range of movement. This makes you more in tune with how you hold yourself and how your muscles react to movement. If one side of your body is especially weaker than the other, performing the exercise slowly can highlight that point and allow you to focus on gently restoring strength to the neglected area. The gracefulness of movement in your exercises will take time, but you will start to see how this will cross over into the way you move throughout the day, giving you more confidence within your body and, I hope, in yourself.

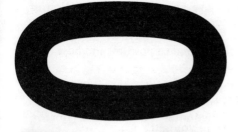

02
understanding your body

In this chapter you will learn:
- how your body works
- the actions of key muscles
- how to improve your posture.

The aim in this section is to give you a basic appreciation of your body: its muscles, actions, functions and movements. There are around 600 muscles in your body. We are going to look at a few of those muscles related to posture, and how they work and affect the shape of your body.

I am sometimes surprised at how much information many people possess about their own anatomy, but then I remember that most people that I encounter have seen a doctor, physiotherapist or surgeon at some point in their life. For almost all of us, including the more active, this is a common experience. Nevertheless, many muscular and postural injuries can be alleviated or avoided with some thought as to the way we move and the way we treat our bodies. Structural fitness exercises like Pilates have a big part to play in keeping us stronger for longer.

This book does not give you the ability to self-diagnose specific injuries; that is the role of a qualified practitioner. However, just looking at yourself naked in a mirror can give you a basic idea of where possible imbalances can be. If you have large muscular shoulders but a tiny weak back, then there is an imbalance. If the latissimus dorsi muscle (the big muscle across your back) is much bigger on one side than the other, this will cause a stronger pull on one side of your body and create an imbalance.

My hope is that this chapter will set the ball rolling for you to find out what your body needs to get yourself into better shape. Through your own quest for improved health or performance, you will research or seek advice for what your body needs. Unless you have a personal trainer/physiotherapist/doctor on call 24 hours a day, then the onus is on you to take responsibility for your health.

One of my old Chinese martial arts instructors explained to me how the medical practitioners treated people in his village. His local doctor would prescribe exercises as part of his medical treatment and send his patients to exercise classes to improve their health. If the doctor found out that the patients were not regularly practising, he would refuse to treat them until they resumed their exercising. Similarly, you must take an active interest in how to heal or improve the health of your body; if not, then accept the consequences and smile.

Muscles

There are three types of muscles in the body:

- Cardiac muscle – this is the muscle found only in the heart;
- Unstriated or involuntary muscles – these are the muscles that can be found controlling the functions of our organs;
- Striated muscles or skeletal muscles – these are the muscles that attach to the skin, bone, cartilage or ligaments. Skeletal muscles are bundles of muscle fibres grouped together by fibrous connective tissue to form an anatomically named muscle group, and these are the muscles on which we are focusing.

Muscles are usually attached by two definite points:

- The **origin** is the name given to the more fixed point of a muscle's attachment.
- The word **insertion** is used for the more movable attachment at the other end of the muscle.

For example, the latissimus dorsi muscle, which covers the middle to lower part of your back, attaches from the spine to the upper part of the arm. The origin is where it attaches to the spine, and the insertion is at the humerus at the top of the arm. To create attachments to the bone, the muscle tissue comes together to form a white fibrous connective tissue. Within certain areas of the body, this connective tissue can become longer to form a tendon. Tendons are used in the body to distance the bulk of the acting muscle from the moving joint, to allow space around the joint for freedom of movement. If you look at the back of your hand when you wiggle your fingers, you can see the tendons moving that connect from your fingers to the muscles in your forearm. Our calf muscles are attached to the heel by the Achilles tendon, to allow space for the free movement of our ankle joint. Muscles can be stretched but tendons lack elasticity and are not designed to be stretched.

These next two pictures show some of the main skeletal muscles of the body.

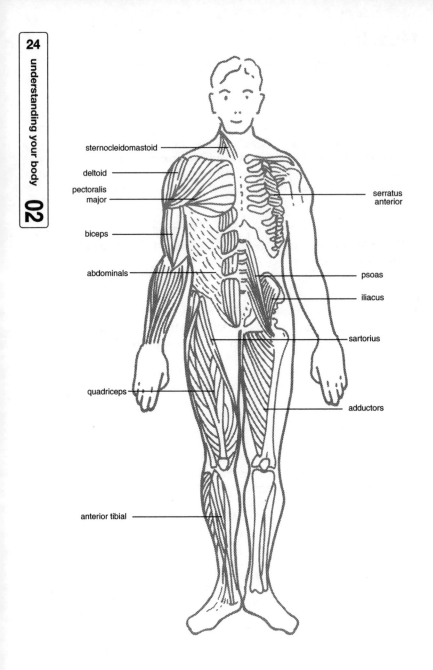

sternocleidomastoid

deltoid

pectoralis
major

biceps

abdominals

quadriceps

anterior tibial

serratus
anterior

psoas

iliacus

sartorius

adductors

anterior view of body muscles

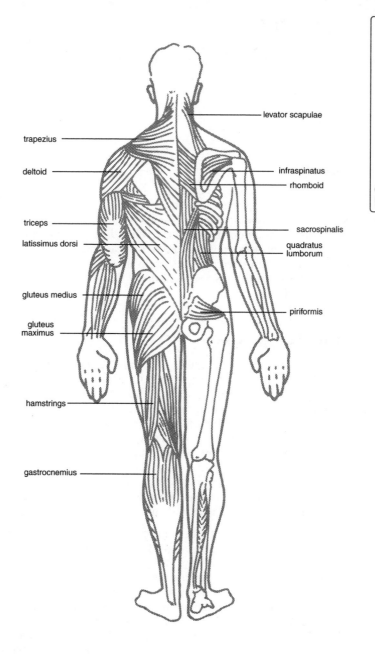

levator scapulae

trapezius

deltoid

infraspinatus

rhomboid

triceps

latissimus dorsi

sacrospinalis

quadratus lumborum

gluteus medius

gluteus maximus

piriformis

hamstrings

gastrocnemius

posterior view of body muscles

Ligaments

Ligaments are the supportive tissue that surrounds most joints in the body where two bones come together. Ligaments are designed to be pliable and strong, to support the movement of the joint. Although ligaments have more elasticity than tendons, they are not designed to be stretched. Most ligaments will tear, if stretched more than six per cent past their normal length.

Nerves

Muscle contractions are controlled by nerve impulses sent by the brain. Most muscles have more than one supply of nerves. When a muscle is stimulated by the nerves, the muscle contracts. The more stimulation the muscle receives from the nerves, the stronger the muscle contraction. A muscle can contract with more energy when stretched and warm. Even at rest there is still stimulation from the nerves to contract the muscles; this gives our muscle its tone.

Muscle partners

Muscles do not work individually; they rely on working in pairs, or groups, to give us our control and co-ordination of movement. The muscle that initiates the movement is called the **agonist,** while the opposing muscle that relaxes to allow this movement is called the **antagonist.** When you bend your elbow to bring your hand closer to your shoulder, you are using your bicep muscle on the front of your upper arm to initiate the movement. In this movement, your bicep is the agonist and the tricep muscle on the back of the arm is the antagonist. If you reverse the movement and extend the arm, these two muscles exchange roles so that the agonist becomes the antagonist.

When groups of muscles work together to create a movement they are described as the prime movers. Muscles that assist in this movement are called the synergists. The term 'fixator' is used to describe the muscles that provide the stability to the body or area while the movement is taking place. If we are bending an elbow and keeping the body fixed, then we will be using fixator muscles in the back to keep our shoulder steady as we move the arm. When thinking about all these different definitions, you start to realize that a single movement of a limb requires an immense pattern of working muscles to perform its task.

Energy

Carbohydrates and fats are the foodstuffs that provide the fuel and energy for the body. Carbohydrates are converted into simple sugars that can combine with other chemicals in the body to create glycogen. Glycogen, which is a form of glucose, is stored in the liver and muscles to provide energy.

When muscles are overworked, they become fatigued and eventually have to stop. This happens because the muscle runs out of fuel and oxygen and begins to build up waste products that make the muscle unable to work. A good supply of blood, carrying the fuel and oxygen, is required to maintain long durations of muscle contraction. Muscles can provide short bursts of power without oxygen, but they soon tire with a build-up of waste products.

Muscle types

When looking at muscles and exercise, we also have to consider the type of muscles we want to build. With Pilates exercises we are building length, stamina and tone into the muscles rather than bulk. If we were looking for short bursts of power combined with great strength, we would focus on high intensity exercises with low repetitions.

Our muscles contain fast twitch and slow twitch fibres. Fast twitch fibres are white fibres of muscle that have a fast speed of contraction. They require a large amount of nerve stimulation and tire quickly, but they provide short bursts of power suitable for sports like sprinting. Slow twitch muscles are red muscle fibres that have a slow rate of contraction. They require less nerve stimulation and are able to maintain their contractions over a longer period of time. This means they are suitable for aerobic (muscles working with oxygen) activities such as long distance running. You cannot create new muscles but you can increase the size and percentage of the type of muscle you require.

A muscle must be worked repeatedly to make it more efficient, or it will soon lose its strength and tone. To build up stamina in our muscles we must provide them with a good supply of fuel and oxygen. This is why we aim to control our breathing throughout our Pilates exercises. Building endurance into our structural muscles will give them the stamina they need to support us throughout the day.

Muscle memory

When you first learned to ride a bike or drive a car, your brain would have been working overtime to deal with all the new movements you had to learn and focus on. Then, after a few weeks of practice, it became easier, and soon afterwards it felt like second nature. With our body's regular repetitive movements, we build up a pre-programmed muscular pattern. These are known as **engrams** or **muscle memory**. Through regular precise practice, we can develop these engrams so that we do not need conscious thought for our muscles to react; it is as if we were on automatic pilot. Think of pianists or typists who do not even need to look at their hands to get the job done. Only with precise, exact repetition is this possible, because practice makes perfect.

Let us look at muscle memory in a destructive situation! We rely on our engrams for most of our everyday movements; we do not have to think when we are walking, running, sitting or driving, we just do these things automatically. Now imagine what would happen if I designed a very bad way for you to move your body, and made you practise all day long so that it became ingrained into your muscle memory. This would mean that, every time you moved around, you were wasting energy and using twice as much effort to perform your everyday tasks. If I also told you that I could sell you a device that could teach your body to move inefficiently, would you buy one from me? Probably not, because you already have one. The average chair is making you slump, tighten your shoulders and weaken your back.

OK, I realise we often have to make the most of a bad thing, especially if we work in an office, but try not to sit for long periods of time, don't use the back of the chair, and try to lengthen your spine and relax your shoulder blades down your back when sitting.

On a more positive note, it is possible to teach an old dog new tricks; it just takes a little time. With regular structural fitness exercises like Pilates, you can retrain your muscles to work with more support and efficiency. Once you become more co-ordinated through your exercises, you will be able to focus more on the breathing that will help to increase your stamina and control. Over time, it will become second nature to move and hold your body with support and strength from your muscles. Remember that muscles do not switch off; they always hold some level of tone (i.e. contraction). That tone needs to be trained in, to maintain a level of support.

Before we move on to the next section, I would like you to ponder this point: Your mind and thoughts control your movements, whether consciously or automatically. Your thoughts are connected to your feelings and emotions. The way we feel in our bodies through our senses and nerves affects the way we feel in our minds. Therefore, we should take care of the way we move, as it can have a profound effect on the way we think.

Actions of the body

The varying movements of the body have their own names. The pictures in the next section describe some of these potential movements.

Flexion: In this movement you are flexing the elbow joint when you bend your hand towards your body. When you bend your body forward, rounding your back, you are flexing your spine.

Extension: This is happening when you straighten your arm and take it to a more extended position. You extend your spine when you push your chest out and lean back, creating a larger hollow in the small of your back.

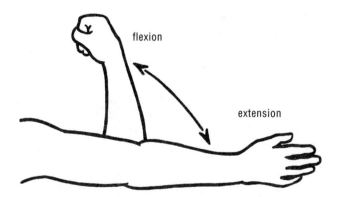

flexion

extension

Abduction: This occurs when you take a limb away from the centre line of your body. In this picture, as the arm moves away it is being abducted from the body.

Adduction: This is when you bring a limb back towards the centre line of your body. In the picture, as the leg is coming back to the centre line it is being added to the body.

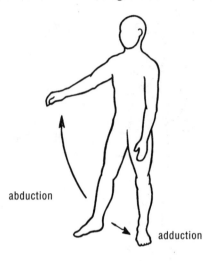

abduction

adduction

Pronation: This is when the palm is turned downwards; if you were lying on your front you would be in a prone position.

Supination: This is when the palm is turned upwards; if you were lying on your back you would be in a supine position.

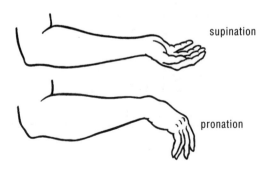

supination

pronation

Medial rotation: As shown in the picture, this is when you are rotating your left arm towards the centre line of your body. If you were to turn your knee towards the centre line you would be medially rotating your leg.

Lateral Rotation: This is when you rotate your right arm away from the centre line of your body. In this action you are laterally rotating your shoulder joint.

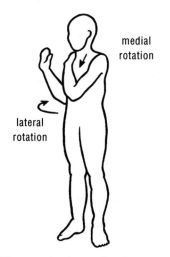

medial
rotation

lateral
rotation

Circumduction: The arm is circumducting as it draws a circle in the air.

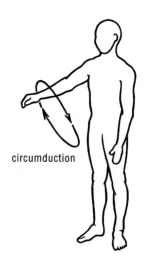

circumduction

Inversion: This is where the sole of the foot is turned inwards with the big toe facing the body.

Eversion: This is where the sole of the foot is turned outwards.

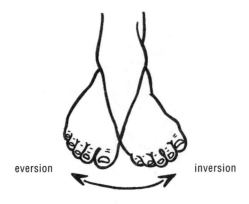

eversion   inversion

Dorsiflexion: This is where the foot is pulled back.

Plantarflexion: This is where the foot is pointed, and it is the only exception for the use of the word 'flexion'; in this movement the foot is actually being extended.

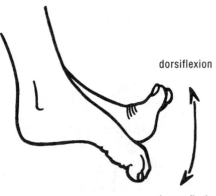

dorsiflexion

plantar flexion

The skeleton

The bones in our body can be divided into four categories: **long, short, flat** and **irregular**.

The **long** bone consists of a shaft with two extremities. The extremities are where the bone articulates (forms a joint with another bone). The shafts of these bones are narrower in their centres and generally larger at the ends, to allow for the attachment of muscle. The long bones are not straight but slightly curved for greater strength. These bones are found in the limbs and are designed to form systems of levers. Some of the bones included in this category are the clavicle, femur, radius and metatarsals.

The **short** bones are designed for strength and compactness. The small bones in the hands and feet make up the groups known as the carpus and the tarsus. Their movement is less, much less, compared with the long bones, and these short bones are tightly held together by ligaments.

The **flat** bones include the sternum, ribs and scapula, and the parietal, frontal and occipital bones of the skull. They are designed to protect or to provide a wide surface for muscle attachments. The scapula (shoulder blade) has 17 muscle attachments, varying from the more delicate levator in the neck to the large trapezius muscles of the upper back.

The **irregular** bones are, as their name suggests, of irregular shape. They do not fit under the above classifications, and in this group are the vertebrae, sacrum, coccyx and palate.

By our late teens to early twenties, our bones are fully formed and we grow no more, although our bones are obviously still living and have their own nerves and blood supply of nutrients. Even though our bones will not grow any longer they still have the ability to repair themselves and increase their density. To increase bone density we need a good supply of vitamins and nutrients, together with increased pulling by the muscles. As with our bones, we cannot create more muscles but we can increase a muscle's size. As the muscles pull more at their attachments, so the bone adapts by increasing its density. Many people have found that performing particular exercises in water is a very safe way of building up bone strength with very low impact on the joints. This can be a great benefit for people suffering from osteoporosis or brittle bones.

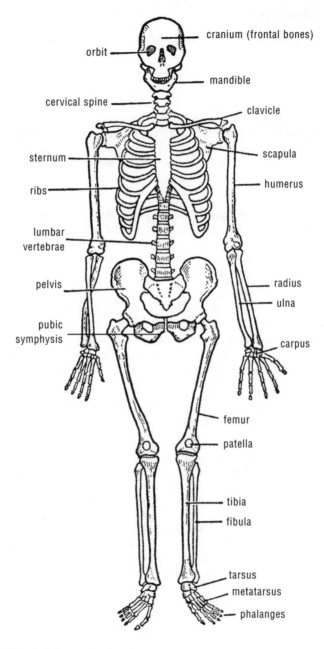

- cranium (frontal bones)
- orbit
- mandible
- cervical spine
- clavicle
- sternum
- scapula
- ribs
- humerus
- lumbar vertebrae
- pelvis
- radius
- ulna
- pubic symphysis
- carpus
- femur
- patella
- tibia
- fibula
- tarsus
- metatarsus
- phalanges

the skeleton, anterior view

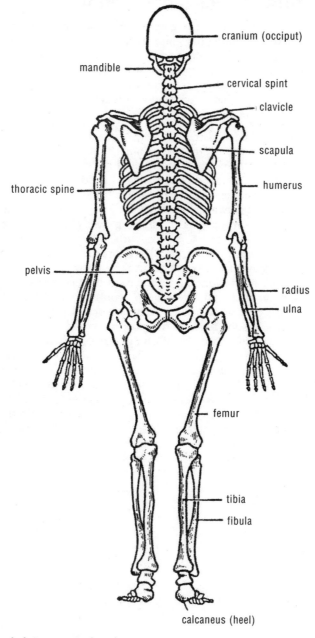

cranium (occiput)

mandible

cervical spint

clavicle

scapula

humerus

thoracic spine

pelvis

radius

ulna

femur

tibia

fibula

calcaneus (heel)

the skeleton, posterior view

Postural muscles and actions

In this section we are focusing on some of the muscles that play a major part in holding the shape of the body and greatly affect the way we move. We do not need to have a detailed knowledge of individual muscles to complete our exercises. However, it is useful to have a basic appreciation of which areas and muscles you are working when exercising and where they attach to the skeleton to create movement.

The **erector spinae** (also known as the sacro-spinalis) is the collective name for the muscle groups that run up the back, extending from the pelvis to the base of the skull. Their actions allow the spine to extend, laterally flex (bend side to side) and rotate. As their name suggests, they keep the spine erect and also bend the spine backwards when the body has to counterbalance a weight at the front – as in carrying heavy boxes or being pregnant. These muscles, along with other deeper layered muscles in the back, stabilize and support our posture, keeping our structural blocks of vertebrae in their upright position. It is the continual relaxation and contraction of these many varied muscles in our back that allows us to maintain our upright spine without tiring. If we relied on only one set of muscles in the back we would soon tire and our posture would collapse. The swimming exercises and the hip hinge exercise (when bending just from the hips) later on in the book give you a strong sensation of working these muscles. Continually bending over with a rounded back to lift heavy objects will weaken these muscles. If one side is weak it will cause the body to bend sideways. Think of these muscles as guide ropes that run down either side of the spine. If one side is slack it will cause your spine to sway to one side. When both sides are weak there is a tendency to become more round-shouldered.

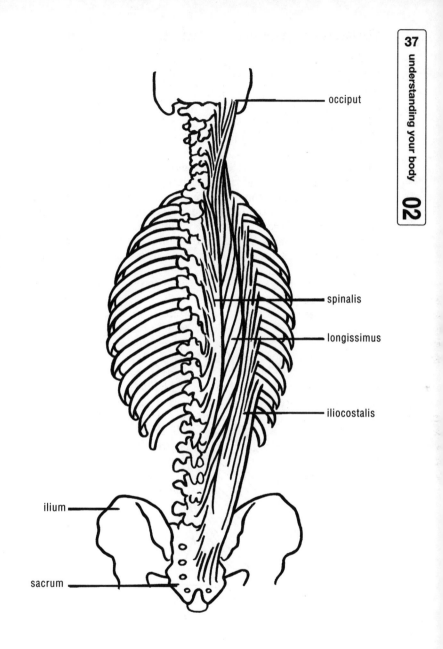

occiput

spinalis

longissimus

iliocostalis

ilium

sacrum

erector spinae (sacrospinalis)

The **latissimus dorsi** is the wide flat muscle that covers much of the back – with 'latissimus' meaning wide and the word 'dorsum' referring to the back. This muscle runs from the six lower thoracic and five lumbar vertebrae as well as the iliac crest of the pelvis. From its origin, it passes over the lower part of the scapula and twists as it inserts into the humerus, just below the shoulder joint. Its functions are to pull the arm down, draw it back and inwards and adduct. You would use this muscle if you were pulling yourself up to climb a tree, or chopping logs with an axe. Part of this muscle's job is to stabilize the shoulder, a weakness on one side of this muscle will cause the shoulder to lift on that side. If the latissimus muscle is not keeping the shoulder down then the lifting muscles around the neck and the upper back will begin to tighten. Pulling the back of the elbow just behind the head while bending over to the side you are pulling to is a good way of stretching this muscle.

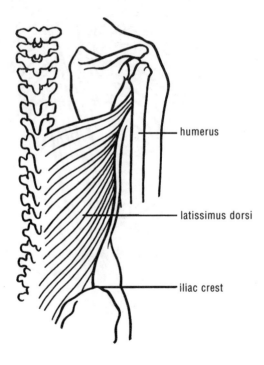

humerus

latissimus dorsi

iliac crest

latissimus dorsi

The **serratus anterior** is a broad muscle that covers the outside of the upper eight to nine ribs from where it originates. It inserts into the medial border (nearest to the spine) of the scapula where its main function is to draw the scapula forward against the ribs, keeping it fixed. With the scapula fixed the serratus muscle can pull on the ribs to aid our thoracic breathing. When lying on your back performing your Pilates exercises you can feel these muscles working as the ribcage expands out to the sides as you breathe in. This muscle is worked when performing a press-up with the shoulder blades held down the back. When there is a weakness in this muscle the scapula will tend to 'wing'; this means that the scapula will stand away from the ribcage, especially when pushing something.

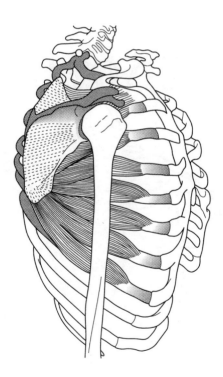

serratus anterior

The **trapezius** muscle is the large diamond-shaped muscle that covers the upper back and neck. It originates at the base of the skull and the cervical and thoracic vertebrae. From there it inserts into the collarbone (clavicle) and the spine of the scapula. Its function is to rotate, elevate and adduct the scapula while aiding in the extension of the spine and flexing the neck to the side. Standing with your arms held out to the side and slowly lifting and lowering the arms will work these muscles. Struggling to lift a weight above your shoulders can highlight a particular weakness within the trapezius muscle. Too much time spent with our shoulders lifted or bending over can cause stiffness and tension in the shoulders; luckily, these muscles are the first place people go for when we are being given a massage. A lovely stretch for this area is the crossed leg stretch described on page 182.

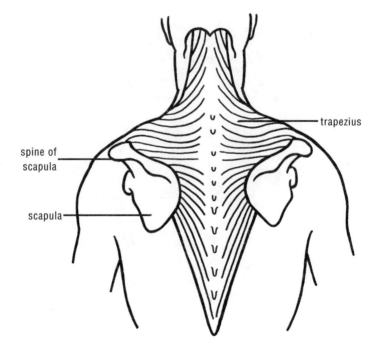

trapezius

The name **rhomboids** describes the parallelogram shape these muscles form in the upper back. They originate from the seventh cervical vertebrae down to the first five thoracic vertebrae, then insert into the inside edge of the scapula. The rhomboids sit beneath the trapezius muscle where they both work together to pull the scapula towards the spine. Imagine if you walked around with your chest pushed out and your shoulders pulled back like an extreme soldier pose. Over time this would cause tightness and tension in the mid trapezius and the rhomboid muscles. When you are performing your arrow exercise with your palms out you can feel the rhomboids pulling your shoulder blade towards your spine. Hugging yourself (which is always nice) with your hands pulling on your shoulder blades is a gentle way of stretching these muscles.

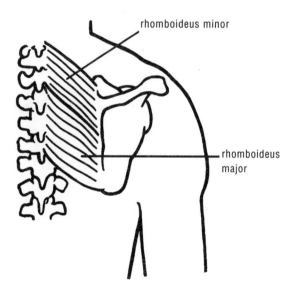

rhomboideus minor

rhomboideus major

rhomboids

The **levator scapulae** is the muscle that assists the trapezius (and others) in lifting the scapula. It originates from the top four cervical vertebrae where it runs down to insert in the top of the scapula. When the scapula is fixed it bends the neck to the side and also aids in the rotation of the neck. Place your right hand on the right side of your head and, without moving your shoulder or your hand, push your head against your hand. Along with your trapezius, you will also feel your levator scapulae muscle working. To stretch these muscles, gently lower your head to your left side, keeping your shoulder down.

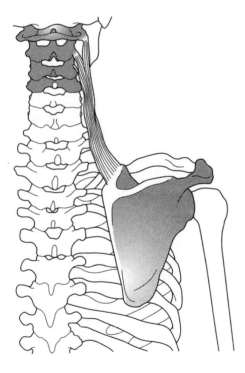

levator scapulae

The **gastrocnemius** is the bunch of muscle that lies superficially on the calf. As the picture shows it has two heads: it originates in the back of the leg just above the knee and it inserts via the Achilles tendon into the heel bone. Its function is to plantar flex the foot, and you feel the muscle working when you stand on your toes. The Achilles tendon is the attachment for the gastrocnemius and is prone to rupture. Warming up, strengthening and stretching the calf will greatly reduce the chance of injury, especially before sports that include a lot of running and jumping. To stretch this muscle, adopt a standing position and take your foot behind your body. Gently push your heel towards the floor until you feel a stretch in the calf.

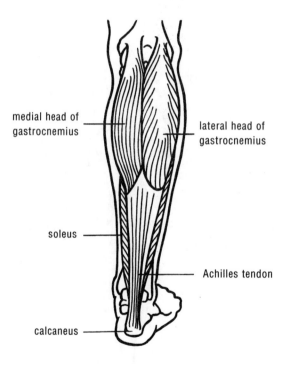

medial head of gastrocnemius

lateral head of gastrocnemius

soleus

Achilles tendon

calcaneus

muscles of the back of the lower leg

The **soleus** muscle sits on the calf underneath the gastrocnemius. It originates on the outside of the leg at the top of the fibula: its job is also to plantar flex the foot and it inserts into the heel via the Achilles tendon. Slowly raising yourself up on your toes and then gently pushing your heel to the ground behind you is a great way of warming up and stretching the calf muscle.

The **hamstrings** are the muscles on the upper part of the back of the leg, comprising the **biceps femoris**, **semitendinosus** and **semimembranosus** muscles. They originate from the bottom of the pelvis and the back of the femur, and they run down to insert in either side of the tibia. Their main function is to extend the thigh and flex the knee. Their strength and flexibility support the pelvis, allowing you to keep your back in a supported position when bending forward at the hips to pick up heavy objects.

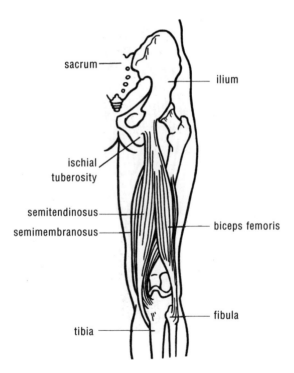

sacrum

ilium

ischial tuberosity

semitendinosus

semimembranosus

biceps femoris

fibula

tibia

hamstrings

The **quadriceps femoris** is a group of four muscles that sit at the front of the thigh, comprising the **rectus femoris, vastus lateralis, vastus intermedius** and the **vastus medialis** muscles. The rectus femoris originates from the pelvis, at the ilium, while the three vastus muscles are attached to the femur. They insert via the patella into the tibia. Their function is to extend the leg and flex the thigh. You rely on these muscles to give you control, especially when kicking, as in football, martial arts and dance. In particular, the vastus intermedius muscle is essential for the final part of extension in the leg, which is required in delivering the last action of a kick. After a thigh injury the vastus intermedius must be carefully strengthened to ensure the balance and control is maintained throughout the full extension of the leg. Pulling the heel towards the buttock with the knee underneath the hip will stretch the front of the thigh.

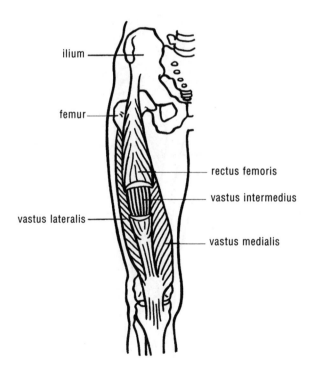

ilium

femur

rectus femoris

vastus intermedius

vastus lateralis

vastus medialis

quadriceps

The **adductors** form part of the muscles on the inner side of the thigh, and it is a group name for the **adductor longus, adductor magnus, adductor brevis** and **pectineus** muscles. These muscles originate from the front part of the pubic bone and the lower part of the hip bone. They insert into the inside of the femur, running all the way down to the knee, and they act to flex the hip, and to laterally rotate and adduct the thigh. When playing sports requiring you to be constantly running around and changing directions, groin strain can be common in these muscles when you overstretch this area. To stretch these muscles, lie on your back with the soles of your feet together, let your knees drop out to the side. To increase the stretch you can gently push down on your knees.

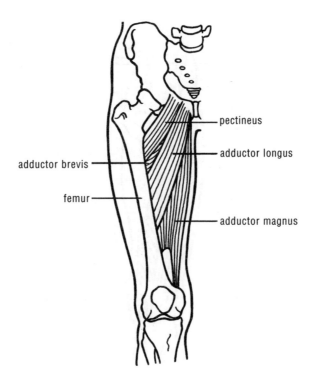

pectineus

adductor longus

adductor brevis

femur

adductor magnus

adductors

The **gluteal** muscles sit on your buttocks, and include the **maximus, medius** and **minimus**. The gluteal minimus lies underneath the two larger muscles and works with other lateral rotator muscles of the hip to open the thigh. The gluteus medius originates on the outer surface of the ilium (outer crest of the pelvis) and inserts into the outer top side of the femur. Its function is to abduct and medially rotate the thigh. The gluteus maximus originates from the back of the ilium, sacrum and coccyx. We need strong and flexible gluteals to maintain the support of our hips and pelvis when walking and running. We also rely on these muscles when we are squatting forward and when we pull ourselves upright from a bent forward position. Lying on your back and gently pulling the knee to the opposite shoulder will stretch around the buttock.

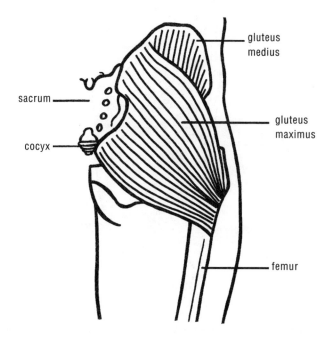

sacrum

cocyx

gluteus medius

gluteus maximus

femur

gluteals

The **quadratus lumborum** is one of the deeper muscles of the abdomen. It originates from the rear iliac crest and the ilio-lumbar ligament and inserts into the lower rib and the four upper lumbar vertebrae. Its function is to bend the spine to the side, aid in respiration and flex the trunk of the body. The quadratus lumborum also acts as a major stabilization muscle of the rib cage; when the muscles on one side are weak, the body can show a slight leaning away from the weak side in the lumbar spine. In Chapter 3, Fixing the Pelvis, we look at the oblique and rectus abdominis muscles in more detail, in connection with the other muscles in the waist.

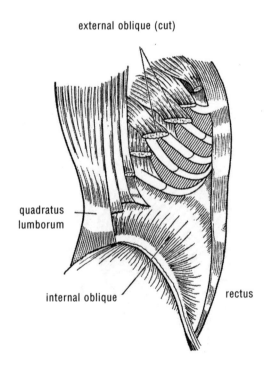

external oblique (cut)

quadratus
lumborum

internal oblique

rectus

the flank abdominal muscles of the right side, intermediate layer

the external oblique has been removed, and the internal oblique is seen exending between the quadratus lumborum behind and the rectus abdominis in front

The **iliopsoas** muscles describe the psoas and the iliacus muscles, which are the main hip flexors of the body. They originate from the front of the lower vertebrae and the inside of the ilium and sacrum, and insert into the top inside of the femur. Their main function is to flex the hip and aid in rotating the hip outwards. Too much time spent with your hips flexed will cause these muscles to become over-tight. Because of their connection to the lower vertebrae, over-tight iliopsoas muscles can cause an increased arch in the lower back, which in time can create a weakness in the lower spine. Performing the quad stretch when you pull the heel towards the buttock will lengthen these muscles, but ensure that you tuck the pelvis towards you and do not extend the back to make this stretch work.

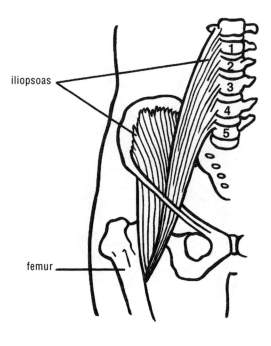

iliopsoas

The **pectoralis major** is the main muscle on the front of the chest. It originates from the clavicle, sternum and upper ribs, and runs across the chest to insert into the humerus. Its function is to adduct the arm and draw it across the chest.

The **pectoralis minor** originates from the third, fourth and fifth ribs and inserts into the shoulder blade. Its function is to draw the scapula downward and inward to the body. When the arms are fixed, both these muscles aid in forced inspiration when you need to breathe more heavily into the chest.

The **sternocleidomastoid** muscle can be felt if you put your thumb just beneath your Adam's apple and turn your head to one side. It originates from the sternum and the clavicle, and inserts into the mastoid process which is just behind the ear. It acts to flex, rotate and draw the head towards the shoulder. When doing a sit-up without supporting the head, this muscle is working to bring the head up. As with the pectoral muscle, it aids in forced inspiration when the head is fixed.

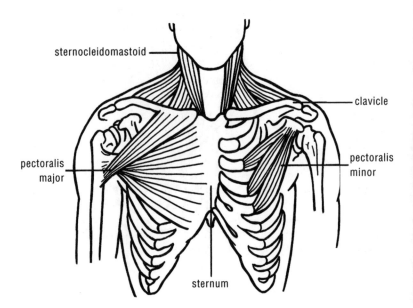

chest and neck muscles

The spine

The spine is an intricate structure that gives our body its versatility of movement. Any injury or loss of mobility in the spine soon restricts our ability to move freely without pain. It consists of seven cervical, twelve thoracic and five lumbar vertebrae; it also includes nine fused vertebrae of the sacrum and coccyx. The top two cervical vertebrae, the atlas and the axis, are specifically designed for the extra movement needed for the skull. The skull sits on the atlas and the atlas slots onto the axis to form a joint that allows rotation and the ability to nod the head. As you go down the spine, the vertebrae become larger as each lower segment has to take more weight and force from the one above. Strong ligaments and muscles hold the vertebrae together. Between each movable vertebra is a cartilaginous disc, which acts as a shock absorber for the spine. These discs contain fluid and can become inflamed, compressed or even slip out of position to cause considerable pain.

Running through the core of the spine is the spinal cord. Nerve endings branch out from this cord in the spine and run throughout our body. If these nerves get trapped by a compressed vertebra, this can cause pain throughout the body.

Keeping your spine strong and flexible is one of the main points of focus in Pilates. Whether you are keeping the spine fixed or moving in your exercises, you are always thinking about its shape and maintaining its support.

For most of us the spine, if seen from the front, would appear to be straight. If you could see a curve from this angle, this would be a form of scoliosis. Scoliosis is a lateral curve in the spine that can be anything from a slight C shape to a more pronounced S shape, and can be formed from birth, by an injury or by a postural weakness. Seen from the side a normally shaped spine will have a series of alternating curves. The lumbar and cervical vertebrae have a forward convex shape also known as lordosis, while the thoracic and sacral areas have a backward facing convex shape also known as kyphosis.

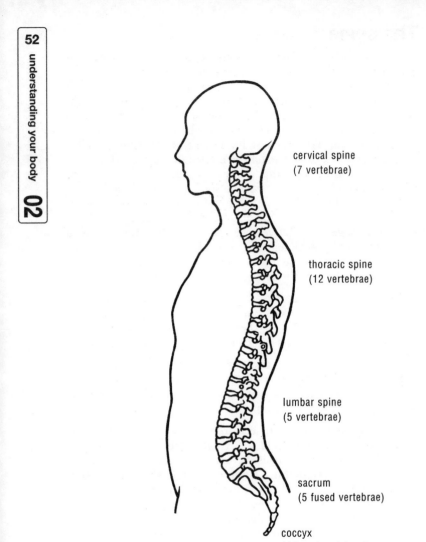

cervical spine
(7 vertebrae)

thoracic spine
(12 vertebrae)

lumbar spine
(5 vertebrae)

sacrum
(5 fused vertebrae)

coccyx
(4 fused vertebrae)

vertebral column

Muscular balance

We have already looked at how muscles work in pairs and with partners to hold and to create movements within the body. We have also already touched on how muscles help to stabilize the body while other parts are moving. For balance to be maintained we need an equal and opposite amount of pull in the muscles. If we think of a child's see-saw and place a heavier child on one end (i.e. more pull) and a lighter child on the other end (i.e. less pull) then the lighter end will be up in the air.

Looking at the picture of the gluteus medius muscle clearly shows that, if the medius muscle was much stronger on one side, it would create a tilt in the pelvis towards the stronger side.

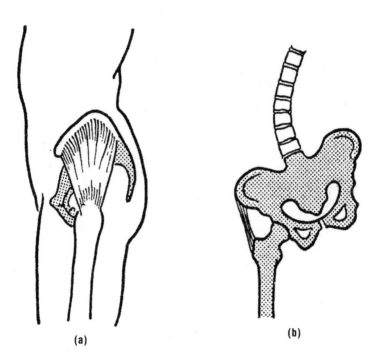

(a)   (b)

(a) the gluteus medius, **(b)** the stabilizing action of the gluteus medius in standing on one leg

Unfortunately, it is not quite as simple as that when diagnosing particular muscle weaknesses and injuries. This is why we need professional medical practitioners with their expert knowledge and use of x-rays, etc., to locate specific muscle problems. However, that does not stop us from looking at more common areas of muscle balance and imbalance.

figure 1   figure 2   figure 3

Posture

When looking at the posture in Figure 1 we can make several muscular assumptions and, if it helps, try to adopt this posture. The shoulders are rounded and the chest collapsed with the chin jutting forward; the abdominal muscles are sagging and the spine is compressed. This position exaggerates the backward curve of the thoracic spine, i.e. kyphosis. Over time, this posture would weaken the erector spinae and the supportive muscles in the back of the neck. This would increase the lordotic curve in the back of the neck, as the chin has to lift to retain the eye line. As the muscles in the back of the neck become slack, the muscles in the front of the neck become tense. Exercises like arm circles, swimming and the arrow will help to correct these muscular imbalances.

When looking at Figure 2, think of a soldier standing to attention: the chest pushed out, shoulders back and legs locked at the knees. In this position, the pelvis tilts forward, slackening your abdominal muscles and tightening your hip flexors. This will increase the pull forward on the lumbar spine, increasing the arch in the lower back, i.e. lordosis. This puts the lower back in a weaker position, especially when loaded with weight from the shoulders. Shoulders pulled back in this position will cause tightness in the mid-trapezius and rhomboid muscles, generally creating tension across the back of the shoulders. Exercises like the scissors and half-splits can help to strengthen the abdominal muscles and increase flexibility and strength in the hip flexors. Exercises like threading the needle, roll down to push up and the heart stretch can help to release the upper back.

When looking for the ideal supportive posture in the body, we must be careful not to create a dramatic change from our normal posture. If you force a sudden change in posture, there is a tendency for your body to overreact and create tension in another area of your body. Over time your Pilates exercises will naturally help to improve your posture, but we must appreciate that this will not happen overnight.

When looking at the better posture in Figure 3 we can see some obvious differences. The chin is parallel to the floor and the eyes are looking straight ahead. The back of the neck is lengthened and the shoulders held down and over the hips. The abdominal muscles are supporting the spine and keeping the pelvis level, while the hips are over the ankles and the knees slightly bent.

Each one of us has our own unique body structure, just as in our fingerprints, but we all share the same basic bone and muscle structures. When looking at how our body performs we should seek to strengthen our weaknesses and maintain our strengths. Remember that there is no rush; take your time to learn the exercises and you will start to see an improvement in your body.

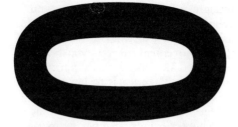

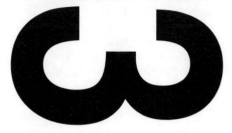

In this chapter you will learn:
- the neutral pelvis position
- how to maintain abdominal control
- the importance of understanding your limits.

With all Pilates exercises you are working from a strong and supported centre. Some of the movements are made with the pelvis in a fixed position, i.e. with your waist fixed, and others are performed with controlled movement of the waist and pelvis. All the exercises are carried out using the supporting muscles around the waist and pelvis. The idea is to have these supporting muscles already engaged before you start the exercise and to maintain their contraction throughout the duration of the exercise. This chapter brings together many of the basic principles that we have looked at earlier in the book. The use of these core supporting muscles is a fundamental part of Pilates; at all costs, even if you have to read this section ten times, please ensure that by the end of this chapter you are comfortable with your **neutral pelvis position, drawing up** and **breathing.**

Neutral pelvis position

We have already looked at body alignment in an earlier chapter and discussed the different shapes into which we get our spine and the varying tilt of our pelvis. Putting your pelvis into a neutral position puts your lower spine into its more natural and supportive shape, in order to produce the least amount of wear and tear in your lower back. It is also providing a strong and balanced foundation for the rest of your body's movements. The next exercise you are about to perform looks at getting you into this position while lying on your back.

Finding it

Lie on your back with your knees bent and your feet flat on the floor, your arms straight down by your sides and your chin tucked in slightly so the back of your neck is lengthened. Now imagine you have a glass bowl full of water resting on your belly four inches below your navel. Lightly pulling on your stomach muscles, tilt your pelvis towards you so that your imaginary bowl of water would spill onto your stomach. Now, gently using the muscles in your back, tilt your pelvis away from you so that the water would spill between your legs. Repeat this exercise slowly at least ten times.

As you get used to this movement, feel what is happening to the shape of your back. When the water is spilling onto your stomach you can feel your lower back rounding and squashing into the mat. As you start to tilt your pelvis away from you, you can feel your back flatten, and then a tiny space appears between the mat and the arch in your lower back (the small of your back). As your pelvis tilts away from you (when your imaginary bowl of water spills between your legs) you can feel the arch in your lower back get larger.

The position on which we want to focus for this chapter is when your imaginary bowl of water sits level on your belly and you have a tiny space between the floor and the arch in the small of your back.

A slightly more anatomical view of this position would be to have the fronts of your hip bones on a level plane with your pubic bone. This is the neutral pelvis position that we are looking for. To get an idea of this, place your fingers in your bellybutton and draw a line two inches straight down. Now draw a line straight out from your centre line until your fingers hit the knobbly bones of your hip girdle. Imagining you have no spare skin on your stomach draw a diagonal line with both fingers towards your pubic bone. In your neutral position those three points of your triangle should be level.

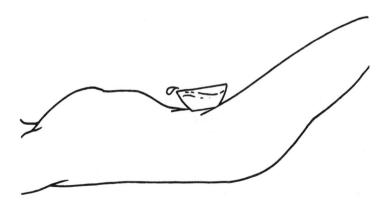

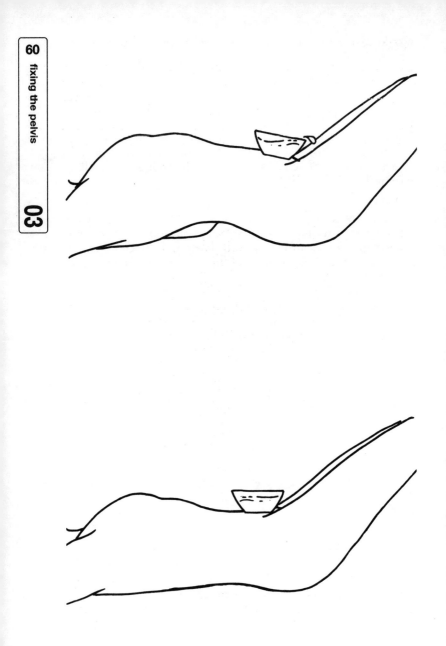

Drawing up

Now that you have found your neutral pelvis position you need to practise using the various abdominal and pelvic muscles to hold it in place. These muscles can be used to hold the lower spine, hips and pelvis in place, or can support the waist and back through a varying range of movements. The sensation in the waist when you engage these muscles is one of **drawing up**.

Abdominal muscles

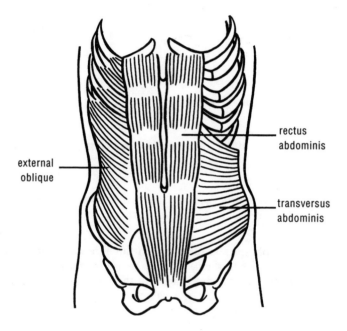

external
oblique

rectus
abdominis

transversus
abdominis

abdominal muscles

The **rectus abdominis** originates from the pubic bone and inserts into the lower ribs and the sternum; its function is to bend forward the trunk of the body.

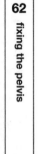

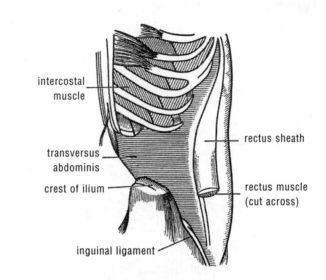

intercostal
muscle

rectus sheath

transversus
abdominis

crest of ilium

rectus muscle
(cut across)

inguinal ligament

**the deepest layer of the flank muscles, transversus abdominis
(after *Gray*)**

The **external obliques** originate from the lower ribs and insert
into the iliac crest. They act to flex, rotate and bend the trunk
sideways.

The **internal obliques** sit underneath the external obliques and
run at right-angles to them. They originate from the crest of the
ilium and the lumbar vertebrae, and they insert into the lower
ribs. Their functions are the same as those of the external
obliques.

The **transversus abdominis** are the deepest muscles of the
abdominal wall and they run around the waist like a thick belt
at right-angles to the rectus abdominis. They originate from the
iliac crest and the vertebrae to insert into the linea alba. The
linea alba is the strong tendinous cord that runs from the
symphysis pubis. When people have very defined abdominal
muscles, you can see this cord running down the middle of their
'six pack', and its function is to compress the abdomen and
assist in exhalation.

As a group the abdominal muscles play an important role in compressing the abdominal organs to expel the foetus in birth and to expel body waste.

The pelvic floor describes a layer of muscle that sits across the base of your pelvis, giving support to the organs.

To give you an idea of how the abdominal muscles and the pelvic floor work together, I should like you to imagine a bucket of water. The bottom of the bucket resembles your pelvic floor, supporting and holding the base, while the abdominal muscles are the sides of the bucket, wrapping around to hold everything in.

To get a sensation of contracting your pelvic floor muscle, the next time you are urinating gently stop your flow a few times. You will get a sensation of drawing up the muscles in your lower pelvic area. Once you are familiar with that sensation, you will find it easy to practise drawing up your pelvic floor.

Lie on your back with your knees bent and put your pelvis in its neutral position. Place the index finger of each hand on your navel. Draw a line three inches straight down towards your pubic bone. Now with each finger draw a line three inches straight out towards your hips. Gently push your fingers into this area and cough; you will feel your adominal muscles pushing up against your fingers. Leave your fingers in this area, gently pushing into your belly, for the next exercise.

Drawing up exercise

Draw up your pelvic floor muscles and pull in your abdominal muscles, as if you were trying to pull your belly button in towards your spine, and your fingers will feel your muscles contract. After a few seconds release and try again, but make sure that you are not tilting your pelvis towards you when you are drawing up these muscles. Remember that your imaginary bowl of water is still sitting level on your belly and you are not spilling the water onto your stomach. Practise this until you feel confident that you can **draw up** and keep your pelvis fixed.

25 per cent contraction

To start off with, the amount of effort we are aiming to use in these **drawing up** muscles (abdominal and pelvic floor muscles) is approximately 25 per cent; in time, as you work at a more arduous level this percentage will increase. To find 25 per cent, first find 100 per cent; you can do this by **drawing up** your abdominal muscles as hard as you can. Now halve the amount of effort you just used and then halve it again. This 25 per cent contraction is the amount that you should maintain throughout all your Pilates exercises.

Breathing

I hope you have remembered to keep breathing throughout the last few exercises. Most people who practise these exercises for the first time find that they are concentrating so hard they forget to breathe and they hold their breath. With Pilates we are aiming to build up stamina in the muscles used, so we need to maintain our breathing throughout the duration of the exercise. The type of breathing used for our exercises is **thoracic breathing**. We did look at this earlier in the section on breathing, but we will go over it again and add all the other techniques you have just learnt. We have to use thoracic breathing throughout our exercises because we cannot relax our abdominal muscles enough to allow the diaphragm to contract. With thoracic breathing we elevate the sternum by lifting the ribs to breathe in, and by doing so we are able to keep our abdominal muscles flat.

Neutral pelvis position, drawing up and breathing

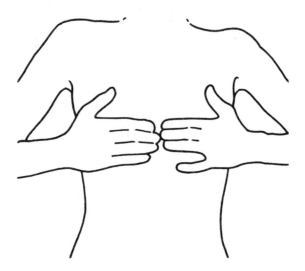

Lie on your back with your knees bent and arms down by your sides. Find your neutral pelvis position, draw up your abdominal muscles and imagine your bowl of water filled to the brim resting on your belly. Place the heels of your palms onto your ribs so that your middle fingers are touching just beneath your breast bone (bra-line or solar plexus).

Keeping your stomach flat push your ribs into the heels of your hands as you breathe in. The sensation you are looking for is that of breathing into your sides, so you can feel your ribs expand outwards. As you do so your middle fingers will slightly separate and then come back together when you breathe out. Make sure you are pushing out to the sides to separate your fingers and not pushing your stomach out. The whole time you are breathing, you are maintaining a neutral pelvis position and drawing up on your abdominal muscles and pelvic floor.

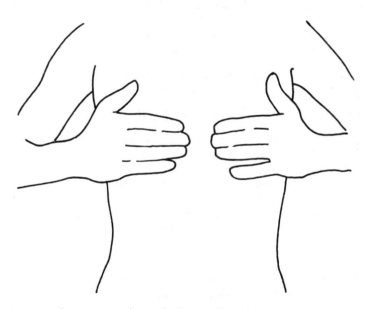

Practise this exercise for at least ten in and out breaths; have a rest and then repeat a further three times. I cannot emphasize enough how important it is to get a basic understanding of all the exercises in this chapter. With your ability to **draw up, find your neutral pelvis position** and **thoracic breathing** you will be able to perform your exercises correctly.

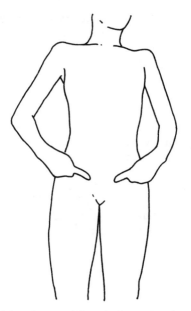

fingers three inches down and three inches out and cough

Understanding your limits

With the next exercise we put all that you have learned into practice to find where your limit of control is. As your strength increases you will find that your ability to perform more demanding exercises will improve along with your body's core strength. Once you have found this limit, do not exceed it. You are training your body to work from a supported centre of strength; if you exceed this limit then you are working from a weak centre and you are training bad habits into your body, as well as running the risk of injury.

To make you aware of where your limit of control is, we must first carefully take you close to that limit. Assume the position from the last exercise, **draw up** and fix your **neutral pelvis position.** Place your index fingers three inches down and three inches out from your navel. If you need to, repeat the coughing exercise described earlier with the stomach muscles relaxed, then **draw up** so that you can feel the contraction of your abdominal muscles. The idea of the next exercise is to feel when those abdominal muscles start to push out. As soon as you start to feel those muscles pushing out, stop the exercise.

Keeping your waist and pelvis in the fixed position, slowly lift one leg off the floor, keeping it bent, then start to straighten that leg; remember that, as soon as you feel your stomach starting to push out, STOP.

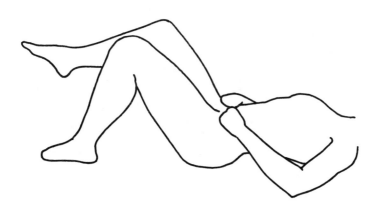

Now, with one leg held straight and off the floor, start to lift the heel and then the toes of the bent leg until you lift the bent leg from the floor (most of you will start to feel your abdominal muscles pushing against your fingers at this point).

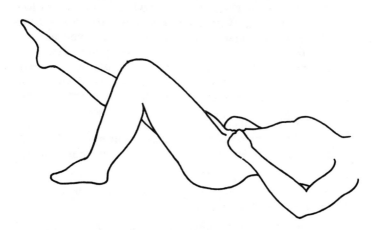

If you are still maintaining your abdominal contraction then carry on until both legs are straight and held just an inch off the floor.

You would be performing this last level, with both legs off the floor, only if you were able to maintain your drawn up position through the previous exercises mentioned in this section of understanding your limits.

The point at which you feel your abdominal muscles start to push against your fingers is the point where you start to lose control of your core muscles. If you were to carry on past this point, your pelvis would start to tilt away from you and the imaginary bowl of water would spill between your legs. With some of the Pilates movements we maintain that neutral pelvis position; with others we maintain just the drawing up contraction of the abdominal and pelvic floor muscles. Never lose that drawing up contraction of the muscles in the waist throughout your Pilates exercises, i.e. do not let your stomach push out and lose the sensation of pulling your navel in towards your spine. Again, repeat this exercise at least five times and this point will be very clear.

Well done for getting through that! We are now going to have a quick recap of the main points.

Drawing up refers to contracting your pelvic floor and abdominal muscles, and maintaining that contraction throughout your exercises.

Neutral pelvis is the position where your pubic bone sits level with the front of your hip bones, and your imaginary bowl of water sits level on your belly.

Fixing your neutral pelvis position is when you maintain this position by drawing up and using your abdominal muscles like concrete to fix and maintain the position throughout a particular exercise. When you are fixing your neutral pelvis position for an exercise, the natural curve in the small of your back remains the same throughout the exercise and does not get larger or smaller.

Thoracic breathing is used so that we can maintain the drawing up of our abdominal muscles throughout our exercises and still breathe.

Exceeding our limits is when we are unable to maintain the drawing up contraction of our abdominal muscles. This will feel as if the muscles are letting go and your stomach is about to push out.

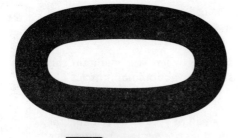

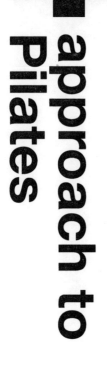

04 approach to Pilates

In this chapter you will learn:
- the importance of regular practice
- about warm up exercises.

Unless you are a professional athlete or a dedicated amateur, you will always find an excuse not to exercise. I very often hear 'I will make time for it next week' or 'there was a great movie on TV' and my favourite 'don't worry, I'll do twice as much tomorrow'. We are all human and I have probably used more excuses than most, but when you realize the benefits to be gained from strengthening your posture and toning your muscles, then it becomes easier to focus on maintaining an exercise routine.

The best way to learn and stay motivated is to book yourself into a Pilates class with a good teacher. There is no substitute for hands-on learning, and the watchful eye of a teacher can reinforce the subtle adjustments needed to perform Pilates. However, this book will give you a good understanding of and grounding in Pilates, and in time you will be able to put together your own exercise routines that suit your individual needs.

Gaining time by making time

When your body is well maintained and the muscles are working in harmony to ensure good posture, you will naturally function more efficiently. This will allow you to stay more relaxed and able to deal with whatever comes your way during the day, and with regular practice you will find you have more energy. Start off with realistic goals that you are able to keep; perhaps three sessions of half an hour a week. You can easily gain this time by going to bed a little earlier the night before.

As the muscles that you are working are structural, it is important to build up their stamina, so little and often is a better goal to aim for. 'Use it or lose it' is a term often used in training the body, and once you start to build up your strength and flexibility, do not let all that good work go to waste. In time you can increase the level of intensity of your workout in order to achieve more noticeable results.

Whether you go to a class or create your own workout, you will start to realize that the time you spend practising Pilates is also a reference point for how you use your body. What I mean by this is: you don't just do your exercises and then go and slump in a heap in a chair, or lift a heavy box using only the muscles in your arms and shoulders. You will start to appreciate that you can draw on the information gained through your exercises to give any movement extra support and stability. You are going to educate your muscles and body in how to support you for the rest of your life. For some, this is re-education and the process will take time as your body adjusts. Stick with it and in time you will not only feel the difference but also see the difference!

General advice

1 Before commencing any exercise routine, you are always recommended to seek medical advice, especially if you are returning to exercise after a long absence or illness. Once you are comfortable with the warm-up exercises, use them – along with the breathing techniques – to clear your mind and practise not allowing other thoughts to interrupt your focus.

2 Make sure your warm-up has been effective. If you feel the warm-up should be repeated in a particular session, then all the better.

3 The great thing about Pilates is that you can work according to how your body feels. If in doubt, start with the easier level before progressing to the next level.

4 It is important to stretch and cool down after you exercise. Continue to listen to your breathing while you are warming down.

5 When you have finished exercising, take the time to lie down and enjoy the extra balance you have put into your body. Remind yourself to walk a little taller, breathe a little deeper and stay that little bit calmer throughout the rest of your busy day.

Warm up

The next four exercises are designed in a sequence to warm up the spine. The first exercise gently flexes and extends the spine; the second keeps the spine lengthened while twisting it; the third flexes the spine from side to side, while the fourth movement aims at keeping the spine supported while stretching and strengthening it. The speed of each exercise is dictated by the speed of your breathing, so keep your breathing slow and relaxed. Use this warm up to concentrate on your breathing and to 'switch off' from the day ahead or the day just gone. For the next 45 minutes while you exercise, your only concern is to make yourself feel better. If you struggle to switch off, then before you start close your eyes and, with your hand on your chest, count to four slowly as you breathe in and to four again as you breathe out. Perform each exercise four or eight times on both sides.

Circle the arms

Stand with your feet shoulder-width apart and your knees slightly bent. Breathe out as you gently round your back and cross your arms in front of you. Breathe in as you bring your arms up above your head, straighten your legs and look up at the ceiling. Open your arms out, palms facing away from you, and begin breathing out as you bend your knees and return to the arms-crossed position.

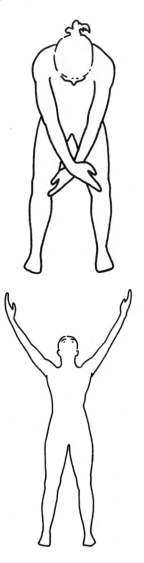

Twist the spine

Standing upright, wrap your left arm around the front of your waist while you slide your right arm behind your back. Keeping your shoulders level, twist to the right as you breathe in and return to face the front as you breathe out. Change hands so that your right arm is in front and your left arm is behind as you breathe in and twist to the left. Keep your spine lengthened as you twist; don't allow any rounding of your shoulders or your chest to push out.

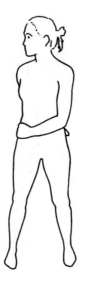

Reach for the sides

With your feet shoulder-width apart, and your right arm down by your side, breathe in as you take your left arm up over the side of your head. Lengthen your left arm diagonally towards the ceiling and then breathe out as you bring it back down so that both arms are down by your sides. Breathe in, reach your right arm up over the side of your head, and breathe out to bring it back down. Try to imagine that you are tightly packed between two panes of glass, so that you can reach only to the sides.

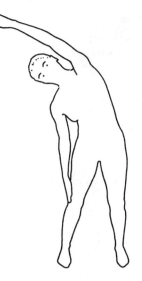

Hinging squat

When you tilt yourself forward in this exercise, you are keeping your spine lengthened while hinging from your hips. Stand with your arms down by your sides and breathe in as you hinge forward at the hips and bend your knees. Bring your arms up in front of you while keeping your shoulders down. Breathe out as you return to standing upright. Make sure that you are not rounding your back or dropping your head.

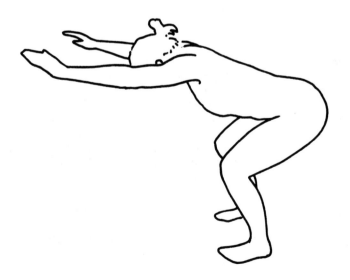

05

level one exercises

In this chapter you will learn:
- how to perform the basic exercises
- to acquire improved strength and flexibility
- the importance of carrying these benefits into your daily life.

Getting started

The exercises for the first two levels are set out in two groups of eight. Together these eight exercises involve the whole body, in order to strengthen the back, front and sides. The strength exercises are mixed up with relevant flexibility movements that will help to lengthen out and release the areas on which you have worked. It is a good idea to read through each exercise a couple of times before you try it. The main point to emphasize before you start any movement is to keep your back supported by drawing up your abdominal muscles. Then you can focus more on your breathing and the alignment of the rest of your body.

Be patient and take your time. Once you are familiar with the first set of eight you can work on learning the second set. Each set of eight is designed to give you a routine that will take approximately 30 to 40 minutes, plus your warm-up time. Once you are familiar with all the exercises at this level you can create your own routine, making sure you feel that you are working the back, front and sides of your body. For example, the shoulder bridge strengthens the back, the arm circles work the front and the side kick tones the sides.

Do not be tempted to do just the exercises you prefer doing, or the ones you find easy. Building up strength in your weaker areas is important in balancing out the structure of your body. Earlier on in the book we have talked about seeking professional help if you are in any doubt about an injury or possible illness. Obviously you should use your common sense about any aches and pains; if something hurts, do not do it. For example, if your wrists hurt, do not do any push-up exercises, but try resting on your elbows; if your elbows hurt, try a similar exercise lying down on your front.

There is no rush, nor even any need, to move on to the more arduous levels of exercises. You may find that the level one exercises are challenging your body enough. On the other hand, you may be able to move on quickly to the advanced movements. Make sure that you go right through each level before trying the next one. Each level holds the basic technique for the level ahead of it, and chances are that you would miss many of the subtleties by heading straight for the end of the book. Remember that, before you start any level, you must have completed and feel confident with the exercises in Chapter 3, **Fixing the pelvis.**

Breathing leg lift

Benefits: Strengthens the waist and back and ensures that you are doing thoracic breathing.

a Lie on your back with your knees bent hip-width apart, your feet flat on the floor, and your head resting on the floor with your chin slightly tucked in, to lengthen the back of your neck. Place the heels of your palms onto your ribcage with your middle fingers touching just beneath your breastbone. Find your neutral pelvis position and draw up to fix your waist. Your hands are on your ribs to check that you are breathing into the sides of your body and keeping your stomach flat.

b Once you feel confident that you can maintain this position, lift your right leg, bend it and hold it there for five breaths in and out before you change to the other side and do the same with your left leg. Ensure that you keep yourself drawn up in the waist with your abdominal muscles pulled in and your pelvic floor muscle contracted.

c To intensify the exercise you can straighten the lifted leg and consider lifting the heel of the foot that is resting on the floor.

Repeat four times each side.

Focus: Keep your waist fixed and your chest down. Remember that, if the muscles in your waist start to push out, you are losing that supported neutral spine position and you must reduce the intensity of the exercise. When you are checking your breathing with your hands, you are aiming to feel your ribs pushing into the heels of your palms and not pushing your chest out.

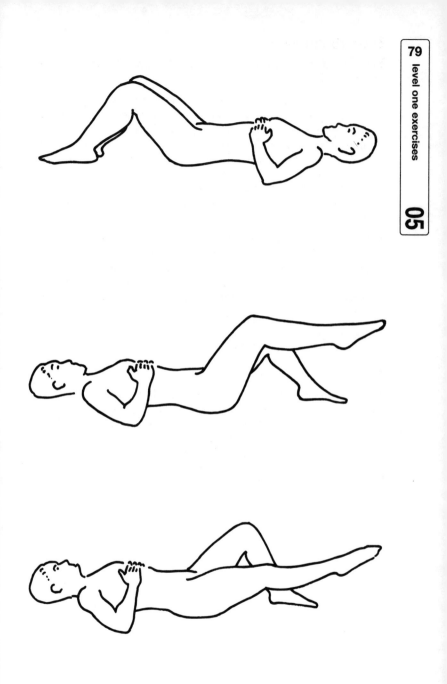

Side to side

Benefits: Rotates the spine, releases the hips and stretches the waist.

a Lie on your back with your knees bent and together, and your feet flat on the floor. Take your arms out into a T shape with your palms facing upwards and your arms level with your shoulders. Keep your head facing up towards the ceiling, and maintain contact between your shoulder blades and the floor.

b Draw up the muscles in your waist and, keeping your bent knees together, slowly lower them over to the right side with the aim of taking your right knee towards the floor. Take at least ten seconds to take your knees over, and just as slowly lift them back up and over to the other side. Ensure that you are engaging your abdominal muscles so you have the sensation of lifting and lowering rather than dropping the knees and then quickly throwing them back up.

c To intensify the exercise you can work with one leg lifted. Change to the other leg once you have lifted and lowered both sides.

Repeat this five times on each side.

Focus: Lower and lift from your centre. As long as you keep your shoulders in contact with the floor it does not matter if your knees do not make it all the way to the floor.

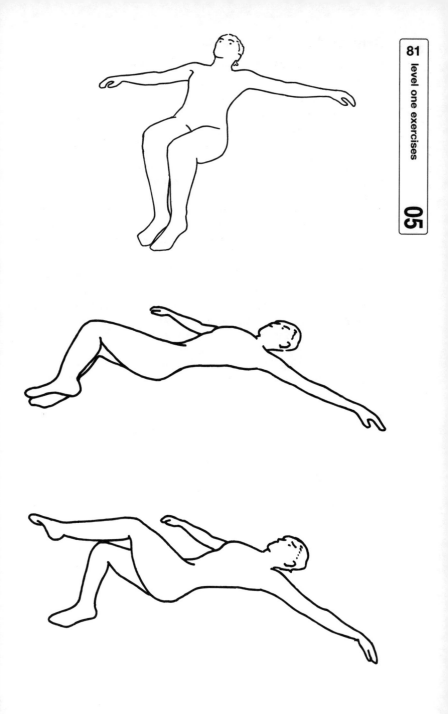

Arm circles and leg raise

Benefits: Strengthens the back, tones the waist and mobilizes the shoulder.

a Lie on your back with your knees bent and hip-width apart. Lift your arms up above your shoulders with your palms facing up towards the ceiling. Draw up and fix your neutral spine position.

b Now slowly lift your arms over your head and draw a circle with your arms out to the sides, around and then back up to the start position. Make sure that your chest stays down and the natural arch in your back does not change shape. Breathe in as your arms go up over your head and out to the sides, then breathe out as your arms come down and back up to the starting point.

c Once you are happy that you are keeping your spine fixed then lift your right leg, bend and hold it for five circles with your arms before you change sides. The most difficult point will be when your arms are up over the head and furthest away from your body. Imagine you have a boiling cup of water filled to the brim resting just beneath your navel. You are maintaining that fixed pelvis position so that there is no movement in the waist and you would not spill a drop of that boiling water.

d To intensify the exercise you can straighten the lifted leg and consider lifting the heel of the foot resting on the floor.

Repeat this four times with each leg.

Focus: Keep your chest and shoulders down. Do not force your arms to touch the floor when drawing your circles. The imprint of your spine into the mat should be the same throughout all of your movements.

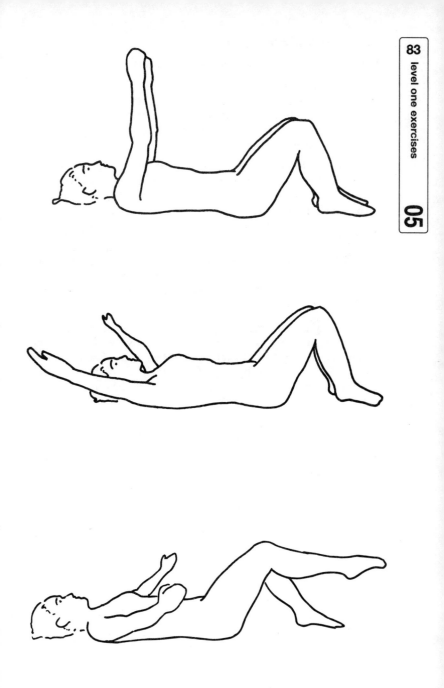

Overhead stretch

Benefits: Stretches the stomach and the chest.

a Lie on your back with your legs out straight and your arms down by your sides. As you take a breath in, lift both arms up over your head towards the mat, point your toes and push your heels away from you. Imagine you are being pulled at each end of your body.

b When you feel the need to breathe out, bring your arms back over and down by your sides. Relax your legs and let your body sink back into the mat. Take a breath in and out and then repeat the exercise five times.

c Starting again with your arms down by your sides, breathe in as you take your right arm up over your head and stretch your left leg out to the side in a diagonal stretch. Breathe out as you return your arm to your side and relax your leg. Perform the exercise on the other side with the left arm and the right leg, and repeat five times.

Focus: Imagine you are a rope and, when you are stretching your arm and leg away from your body, you are being lengthened and pulled at each end. When you relax and bring your arms back down by your sides, let your body sink back into the mat as if you are sighing as you breathe out.

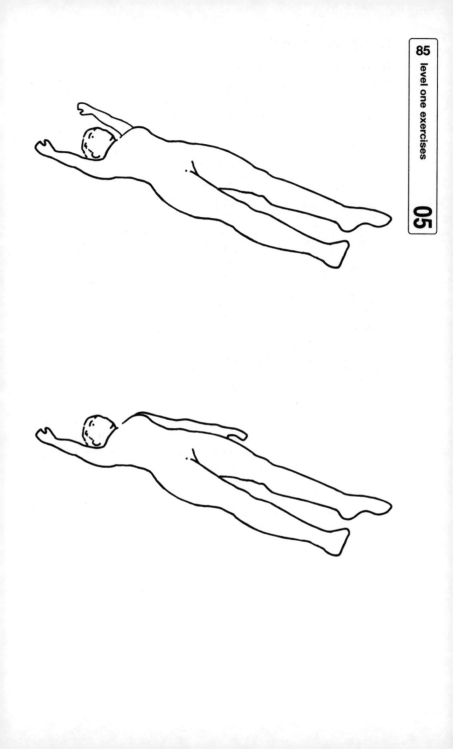

Shoulder bridge

Benefits: Improves the mobility of the spine and strengthens the muscles in the lower back and legs.

a Lie on your back with your knees bent, hip-width apart and your arms resting down by your sides. Have the heels of your feet no further than ten inches away from your bottom. With this exercise it is important to move slowly and with control so maintain your breathing throughout. Starting from your neutral pelvis position draw up and start to tilt your pelvis towards you. You will start to feel your lower back rounding into the floor. Your aim is to gently push each of your lower vertebra into the floor before you peel the next one off.

b Carry on lifting your back away from the floor until your body forms a ski slope position. Keep your abdominal muscles drawn up and do not push past this ski slope position. To take yourself back down use your abdominal muscles to tilt your pelvis towards you and round your lower back slightly. As you return your spine to the mat, touch each higher vertebra before a lower one, trying to round the small of your back into the mat before your bottom, as you return to your neutral pelvis position.

c To intensify the exercise, bring your feet together and move them further away from your bottom. As you peel your spine away from the floor you can take your arms up over your head onto the mat, but make sure that you do not push your chest out past your ski slope position. As you roll your spine back down, bring your arms back over as you round the small of your back into the mat.

Repeat this exercise ten times.

Focus: Initiate the movement of rolling the spine by drawing up your abdominal muscles and slowly peeling yourself away from the mat. If you move too quickly the big muscles in your legs will push up your knees and take over the movement. Visualize your spine as a string of pearls and imagine that you are peeling them away one by one from the mat. Remember that the further you take your heels away from your backside before you lift, the more difficult the exercise becomes.

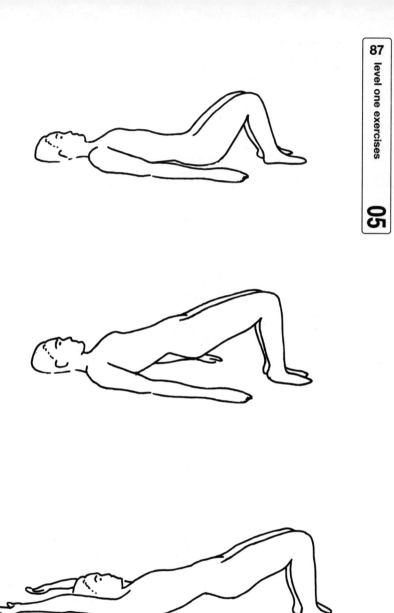

Hamstrings and thigh stretch

Benefits: Improves flexibility in the back and the front of the leg. The hip flexors on the front of the thigh and the hamstrings on the back of the thigh play a major role in affecting your posture and should be regularly stretched. Before you start you may find it useful to have a scarf or a flexi-band nearby to aid with the stretching.

a Lie on your back with both knees bent, then draw up and fix your neutral pelvis position. Without rounding the small of your back into the mat, clasp your hands on the back of your thigh and pull the knee towards you. Hold this position for 20 seconds and then gently straighten your leg and hold for a further 30 seconds. If you are struggling to maintain your neutral pelvis position then use your scarf instead of your hands to pull on the back of your leg. If you are naturally flexible then you can pull on the back of your calf to get your leg further towards you. Repeat on both sides

b Roll over onto your front and draw up your abdominal muscles so that you feel your stomach muscles pulled away from the mat. This will naturally lengthen your lower back and put you into your neutral pelvis position. Bend your right knee, place your hand on your shin and gently pull your heel towards your bottom until you feel a gentle stretch across the front of your thigh. Hold this position for 30 seconds before you repeat it on the other side. You can use your scarf wrapped around your ankle to assist with the stretch if you need it. There should be no crunching sensation in your lower back and your stomach muscles should remain pulled away from the mat.

Focus: Your aim is to maintain a neutral pelvis position in both these exercises, so do not try to get your heel or foot closer towards you by changing the shape of your lower back. By keeping your lower back fixed you can effectively target the muscle groups at which we are aiming in this stretch.

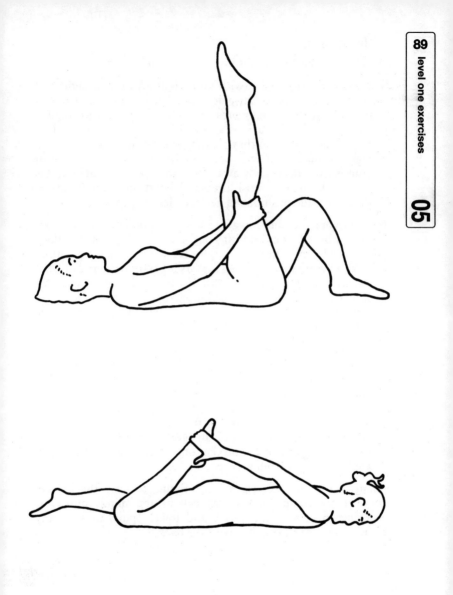

Side legs lift

Benefits: Strengthens and tones the hips and waist.

a Lie on your right side with your right arm out straight and your head resting on it; place your left hand out in front of your chest. Straighten your legs so that your heels are aligned with your hips. Your hips and your shoulders are aligned on top of each other, so they are stacked. Draw up and you will feel the muscles in your waist contract as the right side of your waist pulls slightly away from the floor. Throughout this exercise keep your waist lifted and lengthened and do not let that right side push out to get your legs higher.

b Point your toes and imagine someone is pulling on your foot as you breathe out and lift your left leg as high off the floor as it will comfortably go without losing your start position. Take a breath in as your leg is at its highest point, and breathe out as you slowly lower your leg to the floor. As your leg comes back to the start position, take a breath in before you begin to lift it again. Repeat up to 20 times before you change over to the other side.

c To intensify the exercise you can lift both legs at the same time while keeping your feet together. Your legs will not go as high as in the single leg lift, and you will start to notice that your balance becomes more difficult to control. Your job is to keep your waist fixed and do not start putting lots of weight through your support hand in front of your chest, or start to fall back onto your bottom. Imagine that there is a glass of wine carefully balanced on the topside of your waist and you are not going to spill a drop.

Focus: With this exercise we are aiming to keep the natural curve in the spine. Your strong belt of abdominal muscles is working to control the pelvis and lower spine, to stop any rotation or side flexing in the lower back.

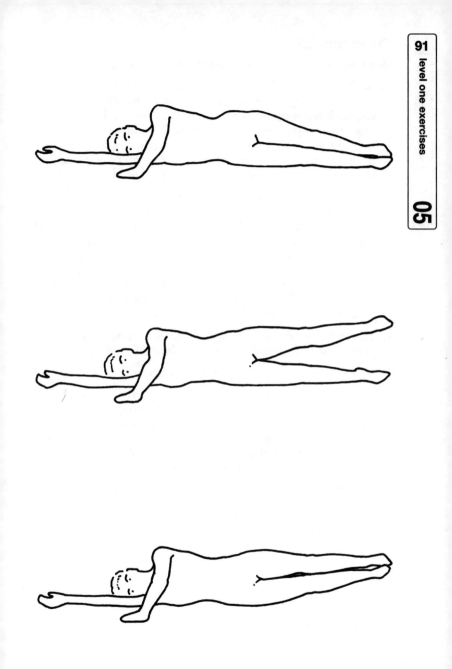

Open a book

Benefits: Releases the hip joints and the waist, opens the shoulders and stretches the chest.

a Lie on your right side and place a cushion beneath your right ear, both for support and to keep your neck in line with the rest of your spine. Place your hands in a prayer position out in front of your chest. With your right leg out straight beneath you, hook your left foot behind your right knee so that your left knee rests on the floor in front of you.

b Draw up and keep your spine lengthened and your left knee on the floor. Breathe in slowly and start to raise your left arm up towards the ceiling. When your left hand is pointing at the ceiling, breathe out as you take your arm behind your body. You are aiming to take your arm back until you feel a comfortable stretch in your shoulder. When you have reached that stretched feeling, take a breath in as you take your arm back up towards the ceiling, and breathe out as you return your hand back into your prayer position.

c The intensity of the exercise will increase in its own time as your chest and shoulders loosen up into the stretch.

Repeat the exercise up to ten times on each side.

Focus: Keep your bent knee on the floor and your abdominal muscles pulled in. There is no need to force your arms towards the floor behind you; just allow your body to release into its own level of stretch before returning to your prayer position. Just as the name of the exercise suggests, imagine that your lifted arm is like the page of a book opening and closing.

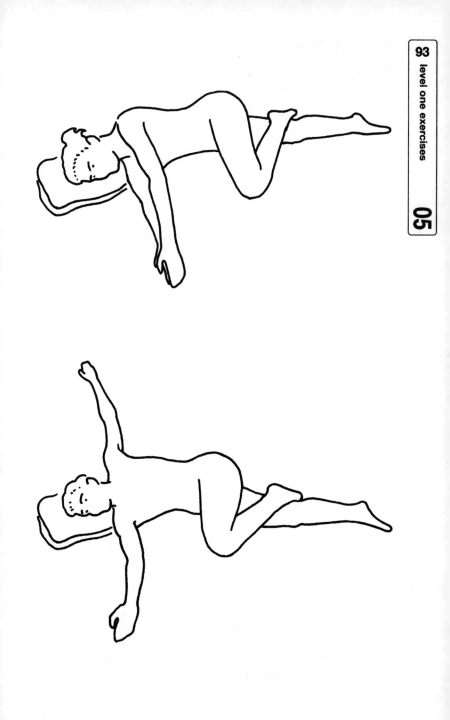

A time to pause

After performing this last set of eight exercises, I hope that you are feeling a little more lengthened and strengthened. I would also hope that you are relaxed and your thoughts are somewhat focused. If not, then do not be disheartened, for as you become more familiar with your exercises you will be able to focus on maintaining the flow of your breathing and your movements. I appreciate that, for the first few times you attempt these exercises, you may be spending more time trying to work out what goes where and which pulls what.

With regular practice you will be creating your own sense of feeling more centred and balanced. This, along with increasing the strength and support in the body, is what we are working for, and the sensation of unity within the body should not be wasted. Take a minute to reflect on how good you feel after your exercise routine, and even if you have to write it on the wall to remind yourself that you can feel this relaxed and strengthened, then do it. The reason I can say this with confidence is because it is three in the morning, I am up writing this book and have just performed these last eight exercises and I feel much better for it.

The job of maintaining and improving your health is not just about knowing the latest exercise craze or buying every workout video available. You are responsible for your own health and you need to find out what your body needs and what helps to make you feel better. If you are one of these super active people who is only happy when running a marathon or climbing the next mountain then you will have to make time for some simple postural exercises if you want to carry on later in life. If you spend all day behind a desk or a steering wheel and complain of a sore back or shoulders, then you have to be doing your Pilates exercises regularly to compensate for those uncomfortable positions you are putting yourself into. The sooner you build a routine of your exercises into your daily life the sooner you can get your body stronger for the challenges and tasks ahead of you.

Disciplining yourself to make time to help your body sounds like a contradiction. Why should I need discipline to do something that makes me feel better? That should be easy to do. Most of the people that I see at the gym or the clinic, regardless of age, tend to fall into two types. One type wants to get more from their bodies and are always talking about their next activity or physical adventure, whereas the other type talks about what they physically used to be able to do when they were younger or when their back did not hurt so much. It is always easier to inspire the first type into maintaining their exercises because such exercises have a definite goal that will allow them to carry out their energetic activities.

For some of the more injured people in the second group, I recommend they perform the same set of twenty-minute exercises three times a day. Most of you reading at this point will start to aim this book towards the bin, but think about it, if you have had back pain everyday for the last five years of your life then an hour a day working towards alleviating that pain and weakness is a small price to pay.

You need to inspire yourself to make the time to get up and keep yourself in good shape. Give yourself your own selfish reasons to feel good about your body and what you can do to help others around you with your new-found vigour. I know that I do not always feel as good as I do right now so I remind myself of this strengthened and balanced feeling when I drag myself out of a warm comfy bed to do some exercises.

When you have finished your exercises and you are feeling lengthened and strengthened, try not to let that good work go to waste. You have, I hope, spent over half an hour working your body into a better shape; keeping your spine supported with your core muscles and gently stretching out possible areas of tightness. Do not then go and slump on the sofa or slouch while you are waiting for the kettle to boil. This will destroy part of the good work you have done. Walk a little taller as if someone is lifting you from the top of your head. If you have to sit, keep your spine upright and use your abdominals to do so, not the back of the chair. Over time you will become more aware of those supporting muscles in your waist, that give you a stronger posture. My hope and my aim is that over time you will not want to put your body into badly supported positions. With your exercises, you are reminding the body how it wants to hold itself so it can work in an efficient way.

Swimming

Benefits: Strengthens the back and the backs of the legs.

a Lie on your front with your hands on top of each other and your forehead resting on your hands. Draw up and feel your stomach muscles lift away from the mat as this puts your lower back into a more lengthened position. Take a little time here to get used to your thoracic breathing in this position; it may feel a little claustrophobic but I promise it gets easier with practice. With your abdominal muscles lifted away from the mat, most of your body weight will be resting on your chest and the fronts of your legs.

b Imagine that there is a glass of wine carefully resting on your lower back and you are not going to spill a drop as you maintain that natural little curve in your lower back. Breathe out as you lift and lengthen your right leg four inches off the floor while keeping the tops of both thighs still resting on the mat. Take a breath in as you hold your leg in position, and breathe out as you lower your leg back to the mat. Breathe in as both legs are on the floor (still keeping your abdominal muscles away from the mat) and breathe out as you start to lift your left leg; then repeat the exercise on the other side. Aim to exercise both legs ten times each.

c To intensify the exercise start with both legs lifted an inch away from the mat and then lift one leg at a time as above.

Focus: When lifting your leg imagine that someone is pulling on your toes to lengthen your leg as you lift. Be careful of lifting your leg too high, and remember your glass of wine resting on your back; you should not feel yourself tilting from one side to the other (no rotating in the spine) or you will spill your glass of wine and we certainly cannot have that! Do not worry if the skin of your stomach is still touching the mat as long as you feel the abdominal muscles pulling away from the floor and your lower back lengthening as you do so.

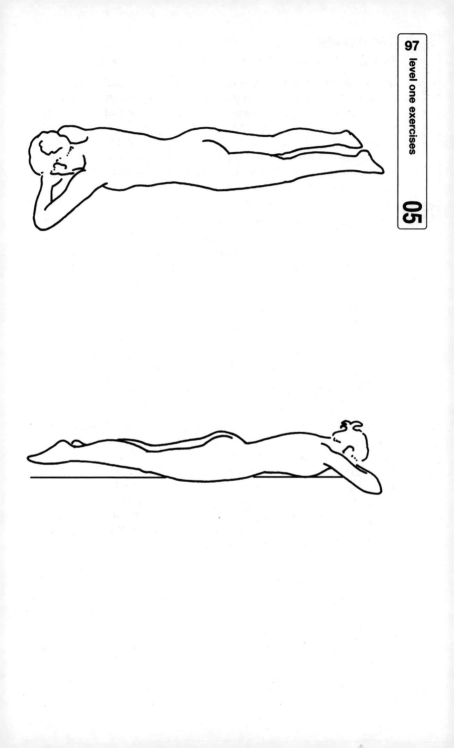

Sit back on heels with diagonal stretch

Benefits: Releases the back and stretches the sides and the shoulders.

a While kneeling down, sit your bottom back onto your heels, bring your chest down onto your thighs and stretch your arms out in front of you as you take your forehead down towards the mat. Relax your abdominal muscles and feel your ribs press into your thighs as you slowly breathe in through your nose and out through your mouth. Stay in this posture for ten breaths in and out.

b From the position of sitting back on your heels, take your right arm down by your right foot. Reach your left arm across to your right side, working your left hand diagonally across until you feel a gentle stretch down the left side of your body. Hold this position for five breaths on one side before you change over to do the same on the other side.

c From your diagonal stretch take both arms down by your feet and rest your forehead on the floor. Let your shoulders come up to your ears as you open up your shoulder blades in your back. Hold this position for ten breaths in and out.

Focus: Keep your breathing slow, and as you breathe out, gently release yourself further into each movement. If you find these movements uncomfortable on your knees then place a cushion under your buttocks to relieve the pressure on your knee joint.

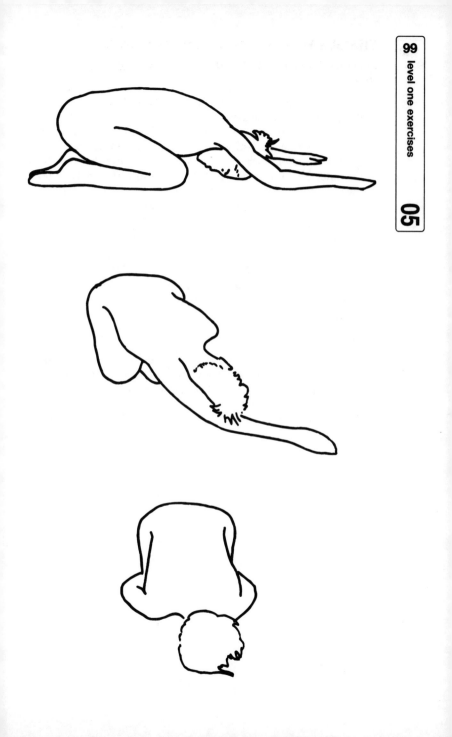

The plank

Benefits: Strengthens the abdominal muscles, shoulders and chest.

a Lie on your front with your elbows and forearms resting on the floor. Your biceps are resting on your forearms and your shoulders are on top of your hands. Ensure the back of your neck is lengthened and your chin slightly tucked under. Tuck your toes under, with your legs hip-width apart. Keeping your shoulder blades down your back, draw up and lift your body away from the mat so that you are still resting on your knees. Hold this position for six breaths in and out before you return your body to the mat. Your aim is to maintain your natural curve in your lower back. There should be no pinching sensation in your lower spine and you will feel that you are working hard to keep your abdominal muscles pulled in.

b To intensify this movement lift your knees away from the mat as you straighten your legs. Keep your breathing slow and controlled, and return your body to the mat after six breaths.

Repeat this three times.

Focus: Imagine that someone is going to use your back as a table and you are keeping your back completely fixed. Your shoulder blades are sliding down your back, and you think of your head and neck as an extension of your table as you keep them in line with the rest of your spine.

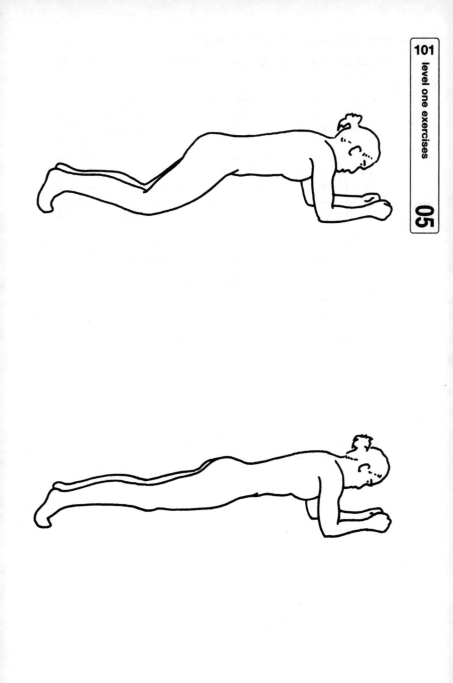

Stomach and thigh stretch

Benefits: Stretches the quadriceps, the rectus abdominus and the stomach.

a If you found the exercise sitting back on the heels more comfortable with a cushion under your thighs then grab your cushion and kneel down with your legs together. Have the tops of your feet resting on the mat and your heels underneath your bottom. Do not let your heels drop out to the side. Start with your palms resting on the floor by your feet. Draw up to support your back and slowly walk your hands behind you as you start to lower your back down towards the floor. Gently take yourself far enough back to feel a stretch in the fronts of your thighs and along your stomach. Hold there for five breaths in and out, and then slowly walk your body back to an upright position.

b If you are naturally flexible in this area then you will need to take the stretch further. Be careful to ensure that you stay drawn up and keep supporting your back, as you will be extending your lower spine. From the position with your hands on the floor walk your hands back until your elbows touch the mat. Continue by placing your arms flat on the floor by your sides before then taking your arms up over your head. Hold this position for five breaths in and out before returning upright.

Repeat this twice more.

Focus: Keep your knees together and on the mat. Your heels should stay underneath your bottom while your spine is supported and lengthened and your abdominal muscles drawn up.

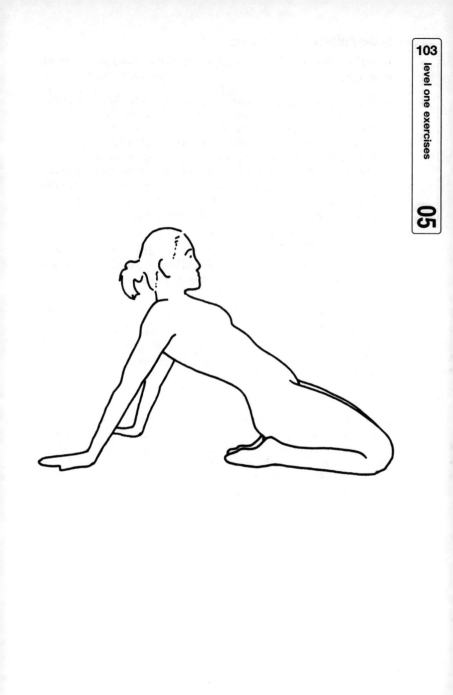

Side raise

Benefits: This exercise strengthens the side muscles of the waist, thighs and hips as well as working the shoulders and the backs of the arms. Care should be taken if you have a weakness in the shoulder as this exercise puts considerable body weight through the arm and shoulder.

a Lie on your right side with your right forearm resting on the floor and your elbow beneath your shoulder; rest your left arm on your left side. Have your knees bent with your feet behind you but keep your thighs in line with the rest of your body. Draw up the muscles in your waist and breathe out as you slowly lift your waist and hip away from the floor.

b The ultimate position we are aiming for is to see a triangle form under the right side of your body; from your armpit to your knees is a straight downward slope. Hold this position as you take a breath in, and then breathe out as you gently lower your hip back down to the floor. Take a breath in as you reach the floor, and breathe out again as you begin to lift.

c To intensify this exercise try taking the lifted position a little higher so that, instead of having that straight line down the underside of your body, you are trying to create a gentle C shape.

Repeat this ten times on each side.

Focus: Keep your shoulder blades sliding down your back and your elbow's start position under your shoulder. Ensure that you draw up before you lift, and maintain that position throughout. Imagine that you have a pane of glass in front of you and your thighs and chest are keeping in contact with the glass as you lift and lower yourself. This will keep your hips and your shoulders aligned.

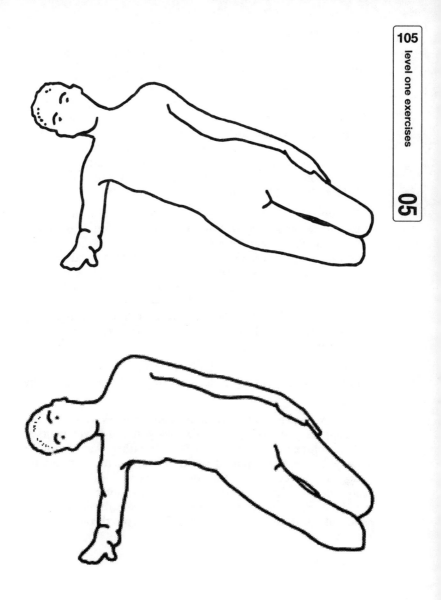

Side stretch

Benefits: Opens up the sides and releases the muscles in the lower back by stretching from the hip to the shoulder.

a From an upright kneeling position on the mat, extend your right leg out to the side. Draw up your abdominal muscles and with your right hand on your right leg slowly lower your right ear down towards your right knee. Imagine that you have a sheet of glass in front of and behind you, and bring your left arm up over your head without twisting your body. Keep drawn up, and breathe in and out for five breaths before you return to the upright start position.

b For this part of the exercise, you may require a block or a telephone book placed down by your bent left knee. From your upright kneeling position, and still drawing up on your abdominal muscles, lower your left ear and left hand towards the floor by the bent knee. If you struggle to place your left hand on the floor, you will need to rest on the telephone book. To increase the stretch, bring your right hand up over your head and stretch your arm over. Hold this position in a comfortable stretch for five breaths before returning to the start position.

c Change your legs over so that your left leg is extended out to the side and your right leg is bent, and then repeat the exercise on both sides.

Focus: By drawing up your abdominal muscles you lengthen and support your lower spine so that you can lower yourself with absolute control into this stretch rather than dropping quickly into an unsupported position. Make sure that you are lifting and lowering into this stretch and not just using your head and shoulders to get you back up. Do not be tempted to lean forward to get closer to the floor; keep the idea of two panes of glass in front of and behind you throughout the exercise.

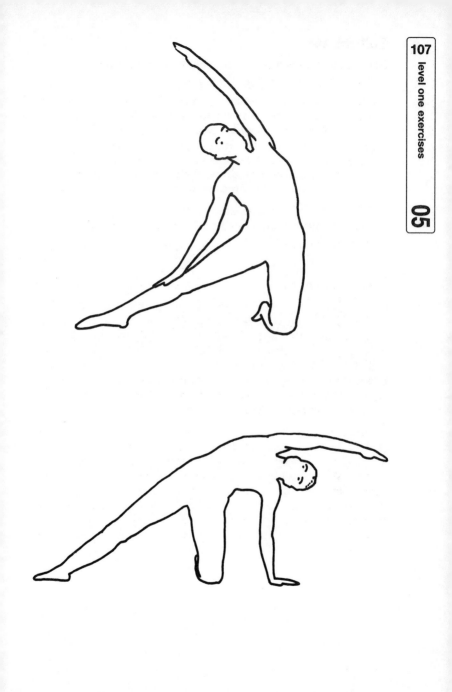

Half roll up

Benefits: Improves abdominal strength and control.

a Sit with your knees bent, your feet flat on the floor and your arms straight out in front of you. Draw up and slightly tuck your pelvis towards you, rounding your lower back into a C shape. With your shoulder blades sliding down your back, gently tuck in your chin and breathe out as you start to roll your bottom and then your lower back into the mat. Keeping your abdominal muscles drawn up, roll back to a point where you can still control the movement from your waist.

b Take a breath in, and breathe out as you slowly raise yourself back to your upright seated position.

c To intensify the exercise try rolling a little more of your lower back into the mat.

Repeat this ten times.

Focus: Your aim is to keep your shoulders relaxed and not be tempted to throw your head or arms forward to get yourself back to the upright position. Your abdominal muscles are controlling the movement of this exercise and, once you have pulled your navel towards your spine by drawing up, you keep those stomach muscles pulled in and do not let them pop up. As your strength improves and the flexibility in your lower back increases, you will be able to roll more of your back into the mat.

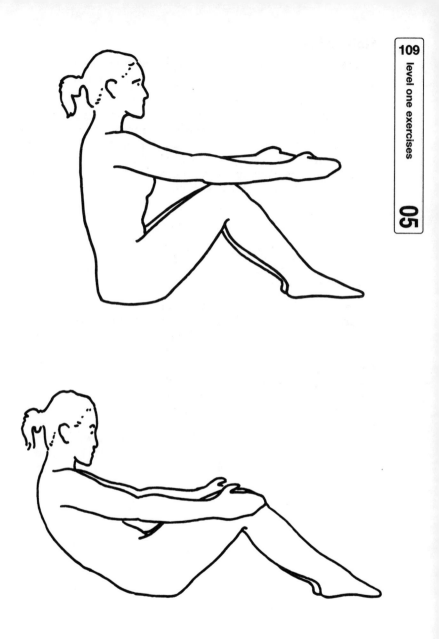

Rolling back

Benefits: Strengthens the abdomen and improves the flexibility of the back while massaging the muscles that run down either side of the spine.

a The idea with this exercise is to create a supported C shape in your back, so that you roll smoothly into the mat and back up. Start from an upright seated position, with your palms on the floor at your sides: your hands are there to control you as you roll back. Tuck your chin down and draw up and tilt your pelvis to round your back into a C shape. Take a breath in as you lift your feet off the floor and roll back as far as your shoulders.

b Keeping your abdominal muscles drawn up and your pelvis tilted towards you, breathe out as you return to your upright position. Try to keep the same distance between your heels and your bottom throughout the exercise, so you are not using the momentum of your legs to get you back up.

c To intensify the exercise place your hands on your shins and, each time you come back to an upright position, lightly touch your toes on the mat before you start to roll back down.

Repeat this ten times.

Focus: The first part of this exercise is very similar to the roll up in the previous exercise. You are rounding your lower spine into the mat and maintaining that rounded back with your pelvis tucked towards you. If you were to let go of your abdominal muscles you would fall back to the mat with a flat back and a thud! Take your time to build up your control and confidence with this exercise.

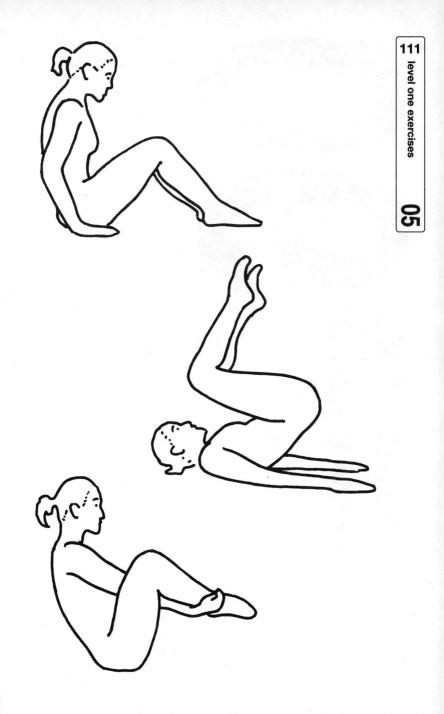

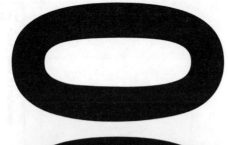

06

level two exercises

In this chapter you will learn:
- a more advanced set of exercises
- how to achieve higher levels of strength and flexibility.

Before you start

These exercises will challenge you further to maintain your control and support throughout your movements. Some of the exercises are adding to the movements you have already learned from level one, so ensure that you are confident with all the exercises at the previous level. Just as with level one, the strength exercises are mixed evenly with flexibility movements. Some of the flexibility movements will require you to maintain a greater level of control in your abdominal muscles. If you struggle with some of the movements at this level, you can pop back to the previous chapter to find a similar exercise that will build up your strength in a particular area. Ensure that you have carried out a warm up before you start these exercises.

Roll down to push up

Benefits: Stretches the back and the backs of the legs. Strengthens the chest, shoulders and waist.

a With this movement, imagine that you are a sheet of wallpaper peeling yourself away from the wall and then being rolled back up the wall as you come back to your upright position. From a standing position draw up and begin rolling your chin down onto your chest as you round your back and carry on taking your head and hands down towards the mat. Bend your knees if you start to find the stretch too strong for your back or the backs of your legs.

b When your hands reach the floor, walk them away into a push-up position, with your hands level with your shoulders and your neck in line with your spine (do not drop your head).

c Take a breath in as you bend your arms and lower your chest down to the mat, and breathe out as you push back up. Repeat the push-up a further three times while keeping your lower back fixed and supported as you go down and up.

d After your four push-ups, walk your hands to your knees and push back on to your feet; slowly restack your body back into an upright position. Your shoulders and then your head should be the last parts of your body to return to upright. Repeat the whole exercise a further five times.

e If you struggle with the full push-up, then come down onto your knees.

Focus: As you are rolling down and up you are controlling and supporting yourself with your abdominal muscles and the muscles in your back. Maintain your breathing throughout, and keep the exercise slow as you feel your back rounding. On the push-up keep your shoulder blades down your back and do not let an over-extended arch appear in your back (i.e. do not let your belly push out).

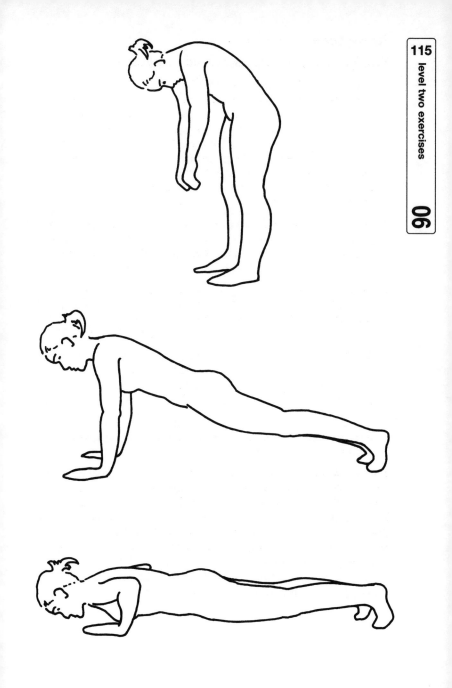

Swimming

Benefits: Strengthens the back and the backs of the legs.

a Lie on your front with your face down and the back of your neck lengthened, legs out straight with your feet hip-width apart, and your arms out above you with palms facing, and with your hands slightly wider apart than your shoulders. Draw up your abdominal muscles and feel your stomach muscles lifting away from the mat; maintain this position throughout the exercise. Lift your face an inch away from the mat while still keeping your chin down.

b Breathe out as you lengthen and lift your right leg and left arm a few inches off the mat, take a breath in at the highest point of your lift and then breathe out as you bring your arm and leg down. Still staying drawn up, breathe in while both arms and legs are on the mat, and then lift and lengthen your left leg and right arm away from the mat as you breathe out. Breathe in as your arm and leg reach the highest point you can manage, and breathe out as you bring them back down to the mat. Repeat the whole movement ten times. Take a 30-second rest and do it again.

c With this exercise, your body weight is resting on the tops of your thighs, your ribs and breastbone. To intensify the movement, lift your limbs and chest higher as you breathe out. Your aim is to keep your body lengthened as if someone is pulling at your head and someone else is pulling at your feet, so there should be no creases appearing in the skin on the back of your neck or your lower back.

Focus: The aim is the same as in level one. Try to imagine a tray of teas carefully resting on your lower back; once you have drawn up your abdominal muscles there should not be even a ripple in any of those cups of tea as you keep your lower spine and pelvis fixed. At first many people struggle with the breathing on this exercise, but if you work hard to get into the breathing pattern of this movement, you will find it helps to keep you going. If you are holding your breath then you are working too hard and need to lower your intensity.

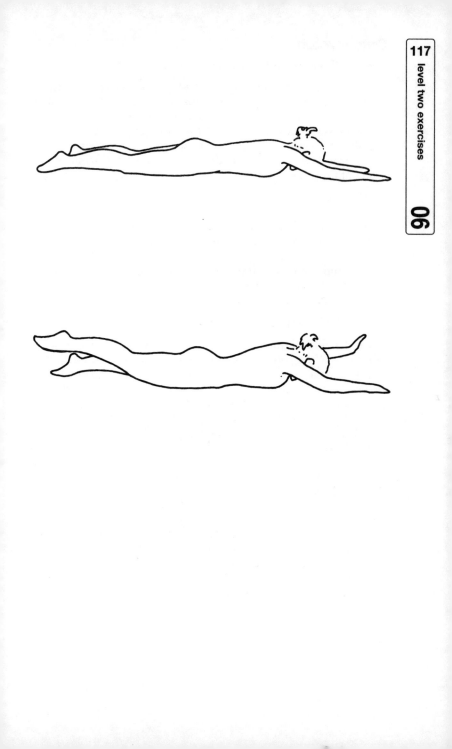

Cats stretch

Benefits: Loosens and mobilizes the spine.

a Kneel on all fours, with your knees underneath your hips and your hands resting just outside your shoulder-width. Draw up and breathe out as you lower your head to your chest and round your back to create a C shape in your back and a hollow in your stomach. In this position your pelvis is tilted towards you and your abdominal muscles are working to maintain this position.

b With the next part of the move the aim is to take your back from a C shape into an S shape. Start to breathe in as you tilt your pelvis away, and lift your head and lengthen your neck away from you as if someone is pulling on the top of your head. Slide the shoulder blades down your back with your abdominal muscles drawn up. Your chin does not push up and there should be no creases of skin appearing on the back of your neck or your lower back.

Repeat this movement ten times.

Focus: It will feel quite natural to keep your abdominal muscles drawn up when you are creating the C shape in your back, but you will have to focus more when you are going into the S shape. Remember that muscles pull, and your muscles pulling in your back are creating the S position, so do not push your stomach out. Think of your head as the point of an arrow as you lengthen your neck, and your shoulder blades as the feathers on the shaft as they slide down your back.

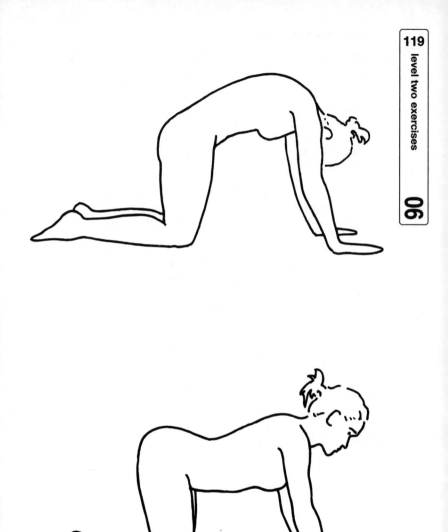

Plank with leg lift

Benefits: Strengthens the abdominal muscles, shoulders and chest.

a Lie on your front with your elbows and hands resting on the mat. Your biceps are resting on your forearms and your shoulders are positioned over your hands. Your chin is slightly tucked in, and the back of your neck lengthened. Your legs are straight out with your feet hip-width apart, and your toes tucked under. Draw up and push down on your elbows to lift your body and the fronts of your legs away from the mat. Ensure that you are keeping a lengthened and supported back, with your shoulders down, your neck in line with your spine and your abdominal muscles pulled in.

b As you keep your whole spine fixed, imagine that two people are using your back as a rest for their chess set as they play. Lift your right foot a few inches off the floor and hold it there for three breaths in and out before you bring it back down. Change to lift your left foot off the floor and hold if there for a further three breaths. After working both legs, lower your body back down to the mat for three breaths in and out, and repeat the exercise twice more with a rest between.

c To intensify this movement try lifting your leg out on a diagonal line, so your foot is out to the side and away from your body. Your bottom should stay down and there should be no sensation of your body weight tilting over to one side.

Focus: Besides feeling the chest and shoulders working, you should also feel the stomach muscles working hard to stay pulled up. Throughout the exercise never let your stomach push out or your head drop. Keep your breathing slow and controlled.

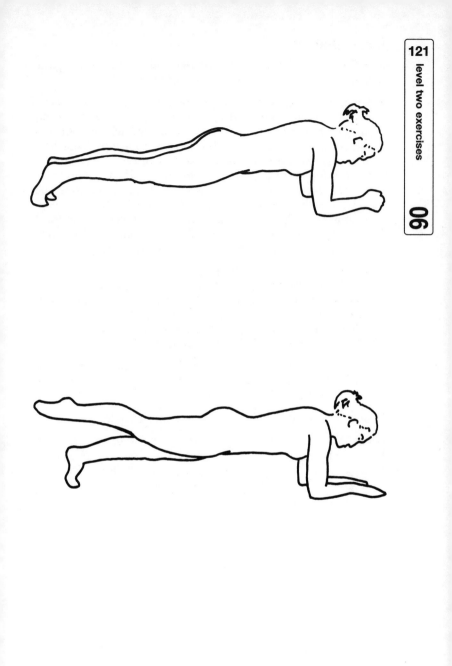

Side kick

Benefits: Strengthens and tones the waist while testing the abdominal muscles to maintain control of the pelvis.

a Lie on your right side with your right arm out straight above your head and your head resting on it; place your left hand out in front of your chest for support. Straighten your legs out so that your heels are aligned with your hips. Your hips and your shoulders are aligned on top of each other, so that the top hip is stacked on the bottom hip. Draw up and you will feel the muscles in your waist contract as your left side slightly pulls away from the mat. Before you lift your legs, imagine that I have placed a fragile pane of glass just in front of your stomach and another behind your back. If your body falls either forward or back you will break them.

b Breathe out as you lift both legs a few inches off the floor. Keeping the lower leg fixed, breathe in as you take the upper leg as far forward as you can while maintaining your balance, and breathe out as you take the leg behind you. Repeat this movement ten times before you bring your legs back down and do the same while lying on your left side.

c To intensify the exercise try taking away the support hand that is resting in front of your chest. Place it on your upper hip or on top of the hand above your head.

Repeat the whole exercise three times on each side.

Focus: You are working hard in this exercise to stop yourself falling either forward or back. Make sure you are not putting much weight through your support hand or falling back onto your lower buttock. If you do that, it means you have broken your imaginary panes of glass.

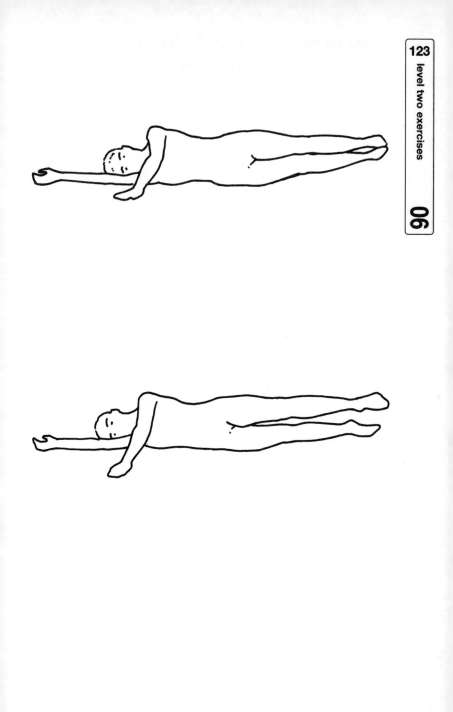

Crossed leg, hip and thigh stretch

Benefits: Releases the muscles around the hip.

a Lie on your back and cross your right leg over your left, with the back of your right knee on the front of your left thigh. With the opposite hand on the opposite leg, place your hands just beneath your knees. Pull your legs closely towards your chest and you will feel a gentle stretch around the outside of your right hip. Hold this position for five slow breaths in and out.

b Bring your left foot down from the previous position and adjust your right leg so that your right foot is resting just above your knee. Straighten your left leg and let your right knee drop out, so you feel a stretch down the inside of your right thigh. Hold this position for five breaths and then repeat both exercises on the other side.

c To intensify the crossed leg stretch, gently rock from side to side as you pull your knees towards you. To increase the opening thigh stretch, slowly pull your foot towards your waist while keeping the other leg straight out in front of you.

Focus: Remember that, with any stretch, you should allow your body to relax gently into it each time you breathe out. You want your body to work with you when you are stretching so do not take the stretch to its limit at first; slowly release into it to feel a strong but comfortable pull on your muscles.

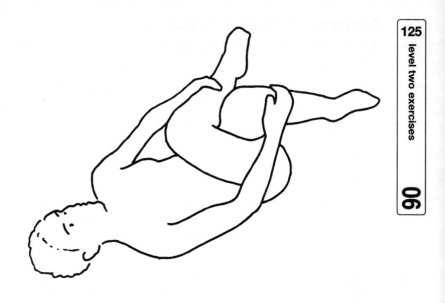

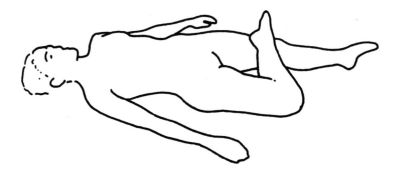

Bent leg scissors

Benefits: Strengthens the abdominal muscles and the thighs; supports the waist and back.

a Lie on your back with your knees bent hip-width apart and your head resting on the mat and the back of your neck lengthened. Draw up and fix your neutral pelvis position. Lift one bent knee and hold onto that knee with your hand as you lift the other knee. Make sure that your abdominal muscles do not push out when you lift both knees. With your knees still bent, get the lower part of your legs parallel with the floor so that you form a right angle behind your knees.

b Imagine that there is a pool of water beneath your feet and that you are going to dip your toe into it every time you lower your leg. Keeping your knee joint fixed, hinge yourself from the hip and breathe out as you lower your right foot towards the floor. Try to just touch the floor with your toes and then breathe in as you return your leg to its lifted position. Repeat the movement ten times with each leg. Have a little rest and then repeat the whole exercise twice more.

c To intensify the exercise, lower your right leg as your left leg is lifting. Breathe in as your legs pass each other at the mid-point, and breathe out as one leg reaches its highest point and the other is at its lowest.

Focus: The natural curve in your lower back should stay the same size throughout the whole of the exercise. Your abdominal muscles stay drawn up and your pelvis remains fixed as you hinge from the hip to create the movement of your leg.

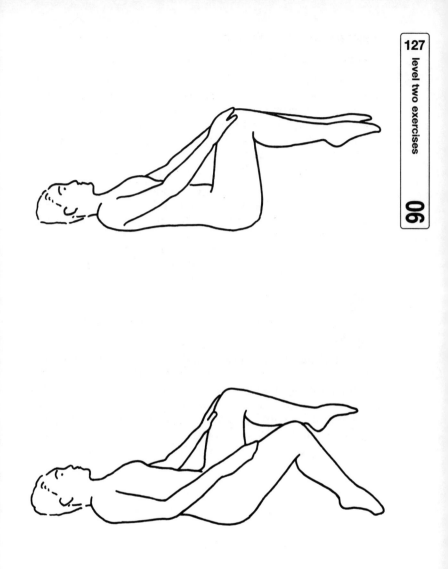

Side to side single leg

Benefits: Releases the hip joints and tones the waist.

a Lie on your back with your knees bent and together, and your feet flat on the mat. Take your arms out into a T shape with your palms facing upwards and your arms level with your shoulders. Keep your head facing up towards the ceiling and maintain contact between your shoulder blades and the mat throughout the exercise.

b Draw up your abdominal muscles and straighten your right leg. Using the control from your abdominal muscles, lower your legs slowly over to your right side. Take them as far as they will go while keeping your shoulders on the mat. Just as slowly bring your legs back to an upright position and over to the other side. Repeat this five times on each side.

c The level of intensity is dictated by the speed of the movement. The slower you go the more difficult it will become.

Repeat the exercise three times with a 30-second break between each set.

Focus: The movement must be slow and controlled from the waist. Do not be tempted to use your legs to get back to an upright position. There is no set breathing pattern with this exercise because this tends to make you speed up the movement. Maintain your controlled breathing throughout, never letting the abdominal muscles push out.

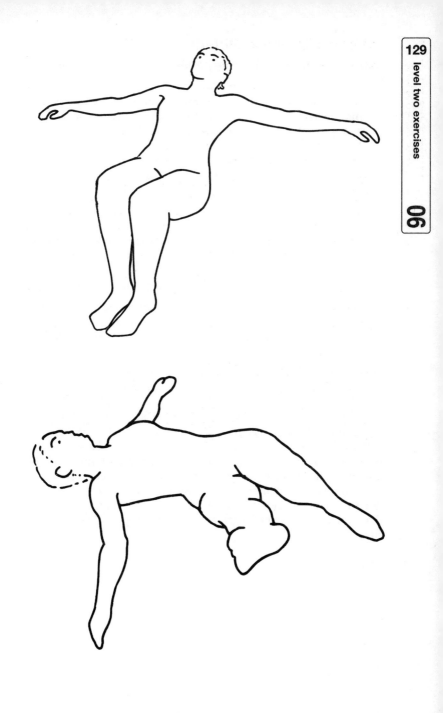

Criss cross (one leg lifted)

Benefits: Strengthens the waist, focusing on the oblique muscle groups.

a Lie on your back with your knees bent, then draw up and fix your neutral pelvis position. Place your hands behind your head and lift your right leg straight up. Keeping the natural space between your lower back and the mat, lift your head and shoulders away from the mat as you breathe out. Twist your spine as you take your right elbow towards your bent left knee. Keeping your head lifted, lower your shoulders towards the floor as you take a breath in.

b Bring your right leg down to the mat with the knee bent, lift and straighten your left leg as you breathe out and lift your shoulders, aiming your left elbow towards your right knee. Take a breath in as you return your left leg to the mat and change to the other side. Repeat this ten times on both sides.

c To intensify the movement, make five lifts on each side before changing to the other leg, and repeat this four times on each side. Take a 30-second rest after the first set of exercises and then do two more sets.

Focus: This exercise is a little more subtle than it looks. The main point to remember is that you are not performing a crunch in this movement (there should be no extra creases of skin appearing on your tummy), but a lift of the body with a little rotation in the spine. The hands behind your head are there only to support your head; try to imagine that you have an egg balanced between your chin and your chest and, if you were to pull your head forward, you would break the egg. You are maintaining your neutral pelvis position, which means you are not rounding the small of your back into the mat. Make sure that you keep the same length between your hips and your lower ribs.

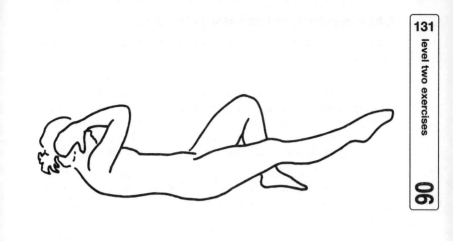

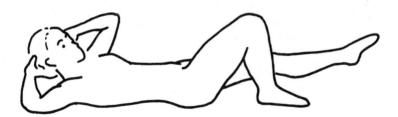

Shoulder bridge with leg extension

Benefits: Improves the flexibility of the spine and strengthens the waist, the lower back and the backs of the legs.

a Lie on your back with your knees bent and hip-width apart. Your arms are at your sides and the back of your neck is lengthened. Draw up and tilt your pelvis towards you as you round your lower back into the mat. Start to peel your spine away from the mat until you reach your ski slope position with your shoulders still on the mat and your chest down.

b Keep your lower spine fixed throughout this next movement, using your strong abdominal muscles. Breathe in as you lift your bent right leg, and then straighten it up towards the ceiling.

c Breathe out as you lower the straight leg towards the bent leg, taking it as low as it will go without losing the shape of your fixed spine. Take a breath in as you bring your leg back to the bent position, and breathe out as you place it back on the floor. Repeat the same movement using the other leg before rolling your spine back into the mat.

Repeat the exercise six times.

Focus: Your aim is to keep your pelvis and spine fixed when you are lifting your leg. There should be no change in the small curve in your back as you move your legs. Your abdominal muscles are working hard to maintain that fixed waist.

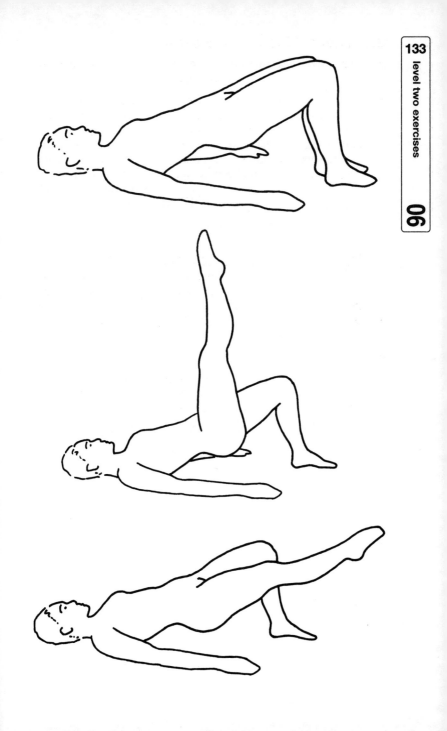

Half-splits

Benefits: Stretches the hamstrings, the hip flexors and the thighs.

a From a kneeling position step up onto your left foot leaving your right knee on the mat. Slowly work your left foot away from you until you feel a gentle stretch at the top of your right thigh. As you relax into the stretch, try to keep your body upright so you are not increasing the arch in your back. This means you are not letting your pelvis tilt away from you and you are able to target those hip flexors more effectively. Hold this position for six slow breaths in and out.

b From the previous exercise, take the weight back onto your right knee. Straighten your left leg, resting it on the back of your left heel. To work into this stretch, tilt your body forward from the hips. Imagine you are taking your stomach towards your thigh, instead of taking your head towards your knee, and this will target the stretch on your hamstrings. Hold this position for six breaths in and out.

Repeat both exercises with your right foot forward and your left knee resting on the mat.

Focus: With both these stretches you are trying to keep the natural shape of your lower back. When you are stretching the front of your thigh, make sure the arch in your back does not increase. When you are stretching out your hamstrings, you are hinging forward from the hip and not rounding your lower back.

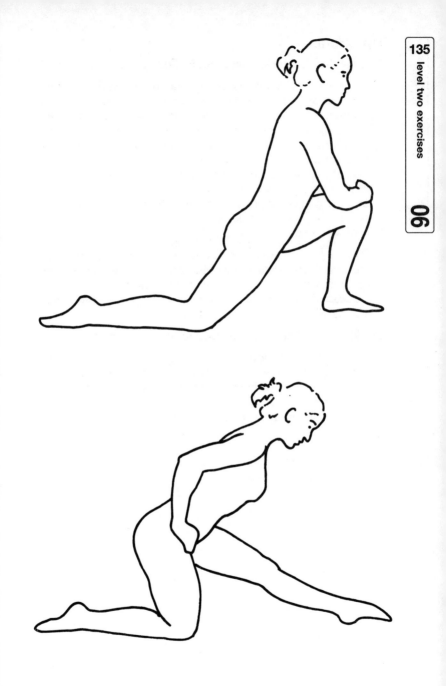

Hip circles

Benefits: To increase strength and mobility around the hips.

a Lie on your back with your legs out straight and place your arms out to your sides. Draw up and fix your neutral pelvis position. Lift your right knee bent to form a right angle behind the knee. With your right knee, you are going to draw a circle in the air. Breathe out as you circle your knee away from your body, and breathe in as you circle the knee towards you. The aim is to make the circle as large as you can while keeping your pelvis fixed. Therefore, your left buttock should not be lifting off the floor and your left leg will remain fixed. Repeat five circles clockwise and then five circles anti-clockwise before changing legs.

b If you have a little more flexibility in your hamstrings and your hip flexors then you will be able to work with your right leg straight. Do not try the exercise with both legs straight if you have to round the small of your back into the mat to accomplish the movement.

Repeat the exercise twice on each leg.

Focus: By keeping your pelvis fixed you are isolating the movement of your leg. As you begin to make the circle larger, you will have to work harder with your abdominal muscles to keep your pelvis fixed. The arms at your sides are relaxed; try not to push down on them for support.

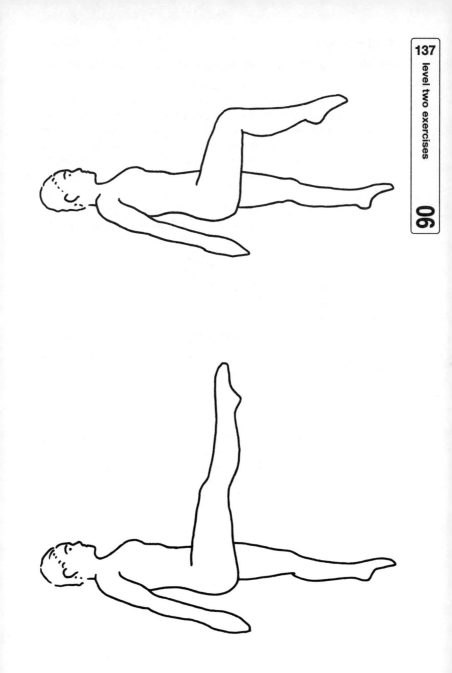

Full roll up

Benefits: Improves the flexibility of the spine and strengthens the waist.

a Sit with your knees slightly bent, heels on the mat and your arms straight out in front of you. Draw up and tuck your pelvis in towards you so that you round your lower back into a C shape. With your shoulder blades sliding down your back, gently tuck in your chin and breathe out as you begin rolling your back into the mat.

b As your shoulders roll into the mat, take a breath in and take your arms up over your head. Breathe out as you bring your arms back over and roll yourself back to your upright sitting position.

c From your sitting position, take a breath in and lengthen yourself up from the waist. Imagine you have a football on your lap and you are going to reach over it to touch your feet. Straighten your legs and reach your hands towards your feet as you breathe out while rounding your back. Breathe in as you restack your spine into your upright sitting position and slightly bend your knees.

Repeat the exercise ten times.

Focus: From when you start the exercise by drawing up your abdominal muscles, you never let them push out. The lifting and lowering phase of the exercise is controlled with the abdominal muscles; there should be no need to throw your arms or head forward to get yourself upright. When you are stretching forward, make sure you are lifting and lengthening your spine before you reach over towards your feet.

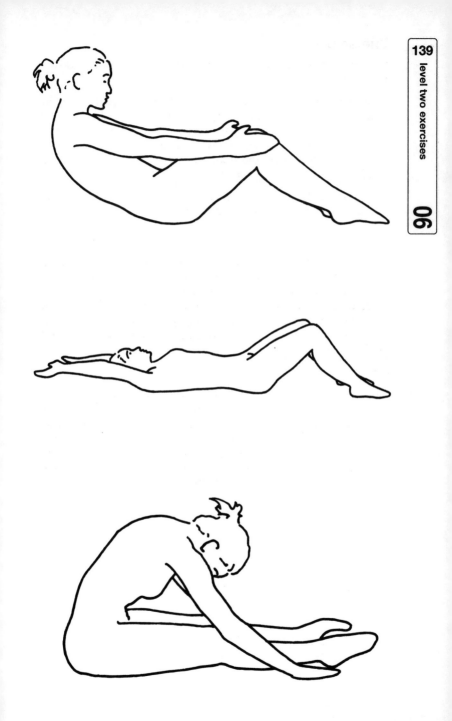

The seal

Benefits: Improves the flexibility of the spine through strong abdominal control and balance.

a Sit upright with your knees bent and slightly apart. Slip your hands underneath your calves and onto the outsides of your ankles. Draw up and tilt your pelvis towards you so that your back goes into a C shape. Stay balanced while you lift your feet a few inches off the floor.

b Tuck in your chin and breathe in as you roll back as far as your shoulders. Make sure that you maintain your rounded back shape to enable you to roll back up.

c Breathe out as you roll back up to a balanced position with your feet a few inches off the floor. Imagine someone is pulling at the top of your head as you lengthen your spine towards the ceiling and sit as upright as you can while still maintaining your balance. Keeping your balance, take a breath in and out, and tap your feet together as if you were clapping your feet. On your next breath in, begin rolling back again.

Repeat this ten times.

Focus: To keep control and balance throughout this exercise you will have to use your abdominal muscles. Especially when you are clapping your feet, try not to take the weight onto your arms, but stay in control from the centre of your body to keep your legs lifted and your body in a more upright position.

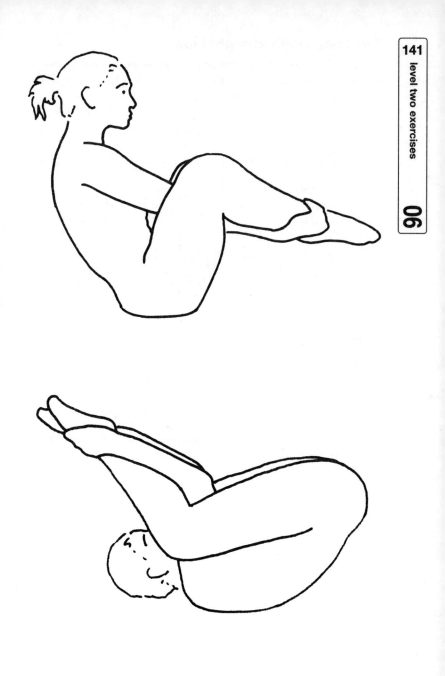

Side raise with straight legs

Benefits: This exercise strengthens the muscles down the sides of your body and also works the shoulders and the backs of the arms. Take care if you have a weakness in the shoulder as this exercise puts considerable body weight through the arm and shoulder.

a Lie on your right side with your elbow underneath your shoulder and your forearm resting on the mat. Your legs are out straight, with your ankles, knees and hips stacked on top of each other. Draw up and breathe out as you lift your waist, hips and knees off the floor. Keep lifting until you form a triangle shape under the right side of your body; from your armpit to your ankles will form a straight downward slope.

b Your aim is to take that downward slope into a gentle lifted curve; there is nothing gentle about the actual movement so go slowly. Breathe in as you lift your left hip up towards the ceiling and reach your left arm up over your head as you stretch your arm away.

c Slowly breathe out as you return your body to your lifted triangle position. As you breathe in start to lift up again and repeat the movement eight times on each side.

Repeat the whole exercise twice on each side.

Focus: Imagine a pane of glass in front of and behind you; it is stopping you moving forward or back. Maintain the drawn up position in your abdominal muscles and ensure you are lifting and lowering with support throughout this exercise; never drop yourself into a position.

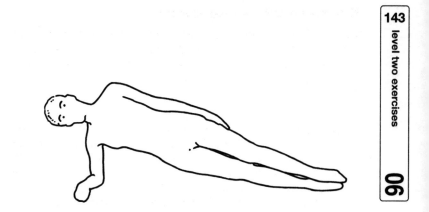

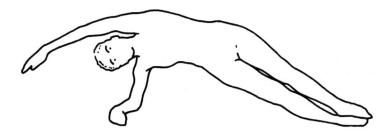

Threading the needle

Benefits: Rotates and releases the spine. Stretches across the back of the shoulders and along the backs of the arms. The head does rest on the floor with this exercise, but the weight is transferred through the shoulder and there is no extra pressure put through the neck.

a From a kneeling position on all fours, place the heels of your palms under your shoulders with your fingers pointing away from your body. Draw up and slide your left arm just inside your right wrist, so that your shoulder makes contact with the floor. Turn your head to look at your left hand and gently rest the side of your head on the floor. The further you push your left arm through, the stronger the stretch will become. Hold this position for five slow breaths in and out.

b This next part of the exercise will increase the rotation of the spine and open up the chest. With the weight of your body resting on your left shoulder, carefully take your right hand up towards the ceiling with the palm facing away from your body. Hold this position for five breaths. To come out of this position, bring your right hand back to the floor, take the weight of your left shoulder and slide your left arm out from under your body.

c To set yourself up to do this exercise on your other side, slide your right arm just inside your left wrist. Turn your head to look at your right hand as you rest your right ear on the floor.

Perform this exercise once on each side.

Focus: If you find the first part of this movement challenging, then there is no need to rush into the second part of the exercise. Remember that, with any stretching, you are trying to relax your body into it. Stay drawn up and keep your breathing slow and relaxed.

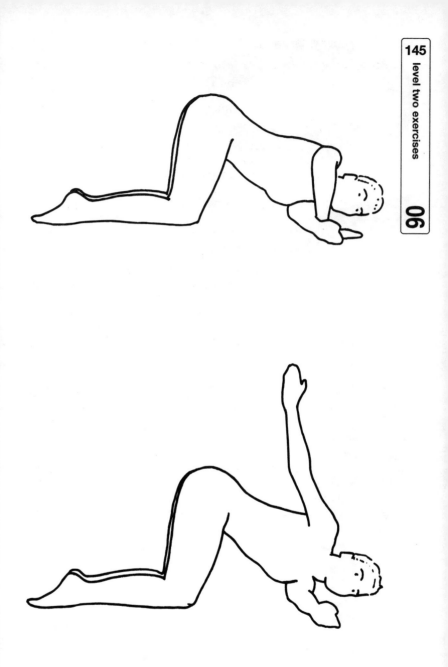

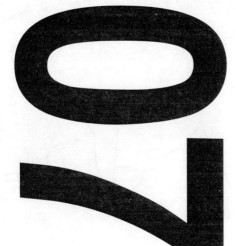

07

advance level exercises

In this chapter you will learn:
- about the role of preliminary exercises
- how to acquire an even higher level of fitness.

You must make sure that you are confident with the level two exercises before commencing work at this level. Many of the movements performed at this level draw on the skills and strength you have gained from the previous chapters. Some of the exercises teach increased levels in the movements that you have already learned and some are new challenges for you to meet.

Although there are flexibility movements in this section, the main focus at this level is strength. If you need some more gentle stretches to mix in with this routine, then you can use the stretches from the previous two levels.

Listen to your body

Remember: What your body is able to do on one day, it might not be able to do the next! Take note of how your body feels; if your body feels like being gentle then go for an easier level of exercises. On the other hand, if you are well rested and energetic, try working to a level that tests you and makes you feel you have worked hard. If you have had a break from your exercises, it is a good idea to go back to some of the more gentle movements described earlier in the book before you return to the more difficult levels. I have added a heading of **prelim exercise** at this advanced level. Ensure that you are 100 per cent proficient at the prelim exercise or exercises before commencing the advanced level movements.

Always warm up before you start, and focus on how your body is moving; listen to how your body is breathing, and maintain complete control and support throughout every movement you make.

Scissors

Prelim exercise: Bent leg scissors

Benefits: Strengthens the abdominal muscles and thighs while supporting the waist and back.

a Lie on your back with your knees bent up and your chin slightly tucked in. Draw up and fix your neutral pelvis position. Lifting one bent leg at a time, take both legs off the floor while still keeping your abdominal muscles drawn up.

b Keeping the natural arch in your back, straighten your legs up towards the ceiling.

c Place your hands either side of your right knee for support. Breathe out as you take your left heel down towards the floor, stopping the heel just an inch from touching the mat. Breathe in as you return your left leg to its upright position. Change your hands over to support yourself around the left knee, then breathe out as you lower your right heel, and take a breath in as you return the leg to upright. Repeat this movement 20 times with each leg. Take a 30-second rest and then do the exercise again.

d To intensify the movement, lower your right leg as you are lifting the left. Take a breath in as your legs cross at the mid-point, and breathe out when they are furthest apart.

Focus: The pelvis and the natural curve in your back stay fixed throughout this exercise; your leg remains straight and you hinge yourself from the hips to take your heel down towards the mat.

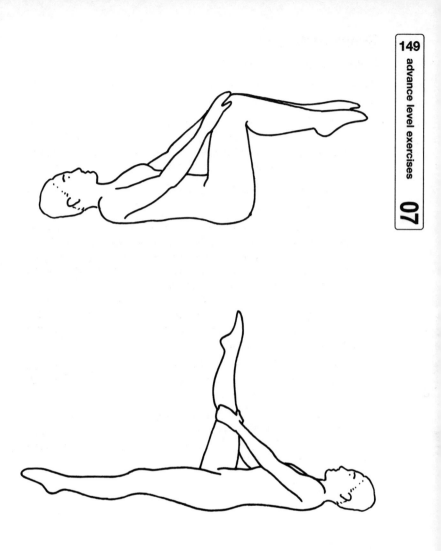

Side to side double leg

Prelim exercises: Side to side single leg, Hamstring stretch

Benefits: Stretches the waist and hips while strengthening the oblique muscles.

a Lie on your back with your arms straight out in a T shape and the palms facing up. Draw up and fix your neutral pelvis position as you lift one leg at a time up towards the ceiling and straighten it out. Keep your head facing up towards the ceiling and ensure that your shoulder blades maintain contact with the mat throughout the exercise.

b Keep your breathing slow and controlled as you lower your legs over to one side. Take them as far over as they will go while keeping your shoulder blades on the mat. Keeping drawn up, slowly bring your legs back to an upright position before lowering them over to the other side. Take your legs over to both sides ten times.

c By slowing the movement down your abdominal muscles have to work harder to keep control.

Repeat the exercise twice with as short a break as possible between each set.

Focus: Make sure that you are working from the waist; if you put too much speed into this exercise you will be throwing your legs up and losing the support in your back. There is no set breathing routine in this exercise because this tends to make you speed up. Every time your legs are raised back up towards the ceiling, your pelvis should be back in the neutral position.

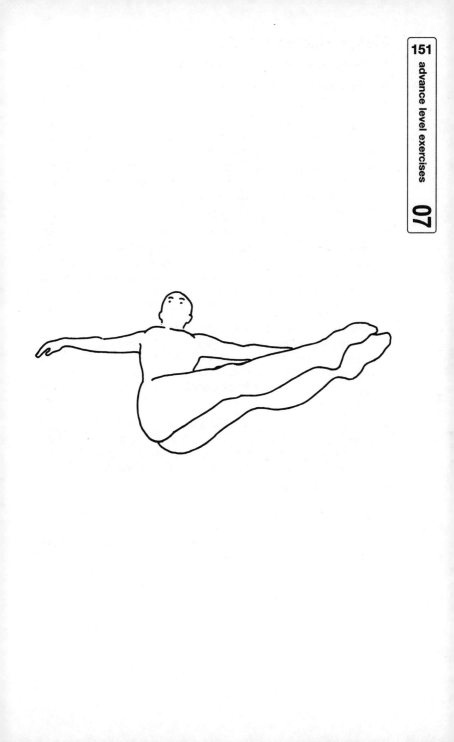

Bridge with hip circles

Prelim exercises: Shoulder bridge with leg extension, Hip circles

Benefits: Strengthens the back and the backs of the legs while toning the waist and improving the flexibility of the spine and the mobility of the hips.

a Lie on your back with your knees bent and hip-width apart, arms at your sides and the back of your neck lengthened. Draw up and tilt your pelvis towards you as you round your lower back into the mat. Start to peel your spine away from the mat until you reach your ski slope position with your chest down and your shoulders still on the mat.

b Use your abdominal strength to keep your pelvis and spine completely fixed throughout the next part of the exercise. Breathe in as you lift your bent right leg, and then extend your foot up towards the ceiling as you straighten the leg. Breathe out as you circle your leg inwards and breathe in as your leg is circling away from your body.

c Aim to complete five large slow circles with your right leg before you swap over to do the same with your left. Once you have completed five circles with each leg, control the lowering of your spine back onto the mat. Make sure that you bring your lower back down onto the mat before your bottom.

d To intensify the exercise take your heels further away from your bottom before you go into your lifted position. Taking your arms up over your head in your lifted position will make you work harder to maintain control while circling your leg.

Repeat the exercise five times.

Focus: Keep your pelvis and spine fixed as you are lifting and circling your legs. Use your abdominal strength to control the tilt of your pelvis as you create a C shape in your back while you are lifting and lowering yourself.

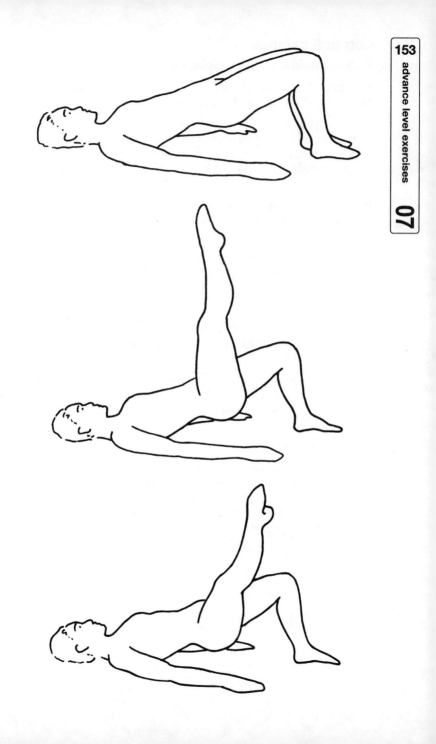

Leg pull balance

Prelim exercises: Seal, Half-split, Roll up

Benefits: Increases abdominal strength and improves the flexibility of the backs of the legs and the spine.

a Lie on your back with your legs out straight, your arms down at your sides and your pelvis in the neutral position. You are going to keep that neutral position until you raise your legs up towards the ceiling; this is a very strong movement to perform.

b Draw up and breathe in as you lift your legs and slowly take them up over your head until your feet touch the mat, and your body is resting on your shoulders and head.

c Holding onto your right shin or ankle, breathe out as you stretch your left leg up towards the ceiling. Take your leg as far over as you can without losing the shape of your body. Start to bring your left leg back over your head as you release your right leg and stretch it up towards the ceiling. Take a breath in as your legs cross over at the mid-point of the movement, and breathe out as your legs reach their furthest point apart.

d Cross your legs ten times before bringing both feet back down to touch the mat. From this position, breathe out as you control the rolling of your body back to the lying position.

Repeat the exercise five times.

Focus: In this exercise the pelvis never tilts away from you. The shape of your back goes from its natural curve into a flexed C shape. If there is a hint of over-extending your lower back past its neutral shape when you are lifting and lowering from your lying position, then you should not be performing this exercise.

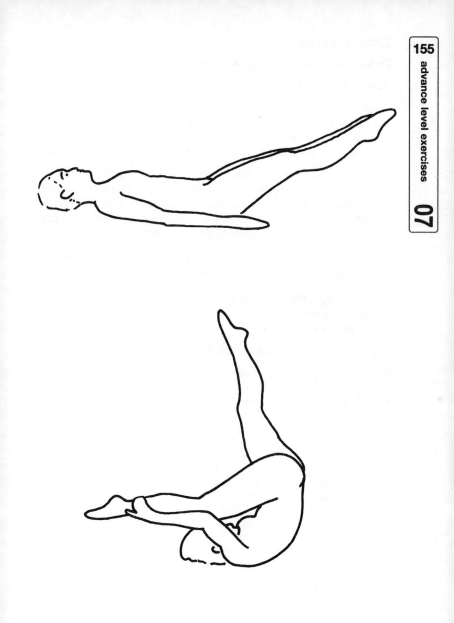

Side lowering

Prelim exercises: Side raise with straight legs, Side stretch

Benefits: Strengthens and lengthens the sides.

a From an upright kneeling position on the mat, extend your right leg out to the side. Draw up your abdominal muscles and, keeping your hands in front of your body and your shoulders and chest down, lift your arms up above your head.

b Imagine that you are tightly packed between two panes of glass as you breathe in and slowly lower your left ear towards the mat, with your arms still above your head. Take the movement as far as you can over to the side without losing control or leaning forward. Breathe out as you slowly lift yourself back into the upright position. Repeat this movement ten times before changing your legs over to the other side and lowering your right ear towards the mat.

c To intensify the movement, stay over to the side for the ten lifts and lowers. The more slowly you move, the more difficult it will become.

Repeat the whole exercise three times.

Focus: You are flexing only your spine from side to side; do not let your pelvis tilt either forward or back. Control the speed of the exercise from your sides.

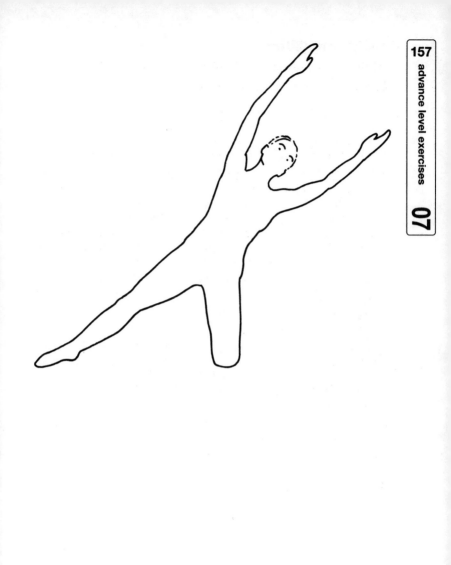

Swimming (lifted)

Prelim exercise: Swimming

Benefits: Strengthens the back and the backs of the legs.

a Lie face down on your front with the back of your neck lengthened, your legs out straight with your feet hip-width apart, and your arms up above your head, palms facing, and your hands slightly wider apart than your shoulders. Draw up your abdominals and feel your stomach muscles lifting away from the mat. Without pushing your stomach out, lift your head, legs and arms an inch off the mat. You should be resting on your chest and the tops of your thighs.

b Breathe out as you lengthen and lift your left arm and your right leg a further few inches off the mat. Take a breath in at the highest point of your lift, and breathe out as you lower yourself back down to the starting height. Breathe in as your limbs are at their lowest point, and breathe out as you lift your right arm and your left leg. Repeat this 12 times on both sides; take a 30-second rest and do the same again.

c To intensify this exercise, perform the lifting and lowering movements very quickly, while still maintaining your fixed waist position. The breathing will not be in time with the movement, so keep your breathing slow, and count 12 breaths in and out before taking a rest.

Focus: Imagine that someone has put a spirit level on your lower back and, every time he sees the little bubble move, you have to give him some money. You are isolating the movements in your arms and legs, so except for your breathing the body should remain fixed.

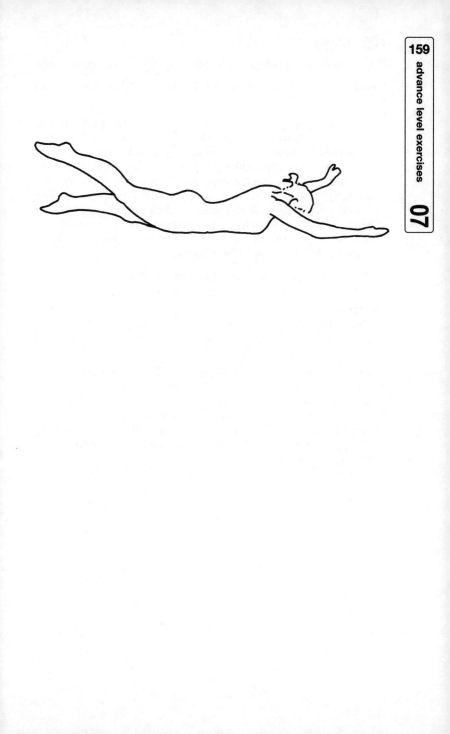

Hip hinge

Prelim exercises: Half-splits, Swimming (lifted), Hinging squats

Benefits: Strengthens the back and legs. Stretches the backs of the legs and improves balance.

a Stand upright with your pelvis in its neutral position and your arms down by your sides. Draw up and slowly bend forwards so that you are hinging yourself from your hip joints and not rounding your spine. Keeping your legs straight, hinge yourself forward until you feel a comfortable stretch in your hamstrings, and hold this position for five breaths. Keeping your abdominal muscles drawn up, lift your body back to its upright position. Repeat the movement, and if it is comfortable try working the stretch a little further as you slowly breathe for five breaths.

b To increase the intensity of the exercise, raise your arms up so that they are in line with your body. This puts more weight through your back and tests you further to keep your lengthened and supported spine. Bring your arms back to your sides after five breaths and complete the whole exercise once more.

Focus: Your aim over time is to keep the upper part of your body parallel to the floor so that your back could almost be used as a table, without any rounding of the spine. Keep the back of your neck lengthened; even dropping your head is enough to start your shoulders rounding. When you pull your arms up, make sure your chest and shoulders stay down; if they push out you will over-arch the back.

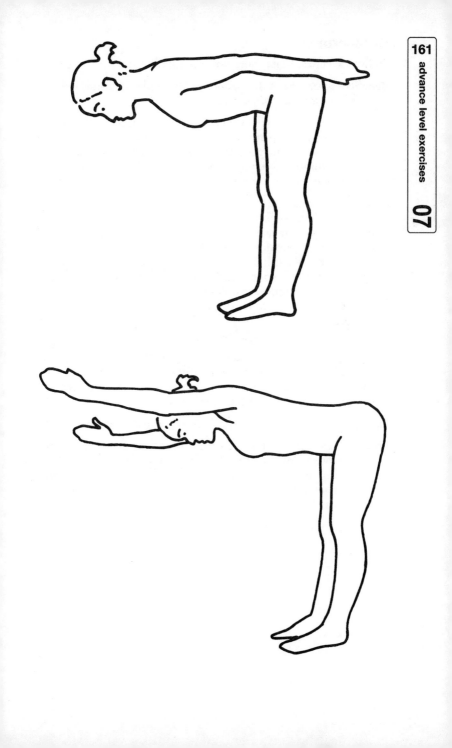

Criss cross

Prelim exercises: Criss cross (one leg lifted)

Benefits: Strengthens the abdominals while focusing on the oblique muscle groups.

a Lie on your back with your knees bent and hip-width apart. Draw up and fix your neutral pelvis position. Lift your head without tucking in your chin, and place your hands behind you for support. Keeping your neutral position lift both bent legs off the mat.

b Breathe out as you extend your right leg and lift your head and shoulders. Twist your spine as you take your right elbow towards your left knee. Breathe in as you return your right leg to its original position, and lower your shoulders to the floor with your head still lifted. Breathe out and extend your left leg as you lift your head and shoulders while twisting towards your right knee. Breathe in as you lower your leg, and repeat this ten times on each side.

c To intensify the exercise, lift your head and chest higher towards the ceiling. Take your right leg out as your left leg is coming back in, and rotate your spine to your left leg as it comes back to its bent position. Breathe in as your knees pass each other at the mid-point of the exercise, and breathe out as one leg extends and the other is bent.

Take a 30-second rest between each set, and repeat three times.

Focus: Remember that this is not a crunch exercise so do not pull your head down onto your chest. Keep that natural little arch in your lower back so that you can maintain the length between your hips and lower ribs. You are aiming your chest and nose up at the ceiling before you put in the twist.

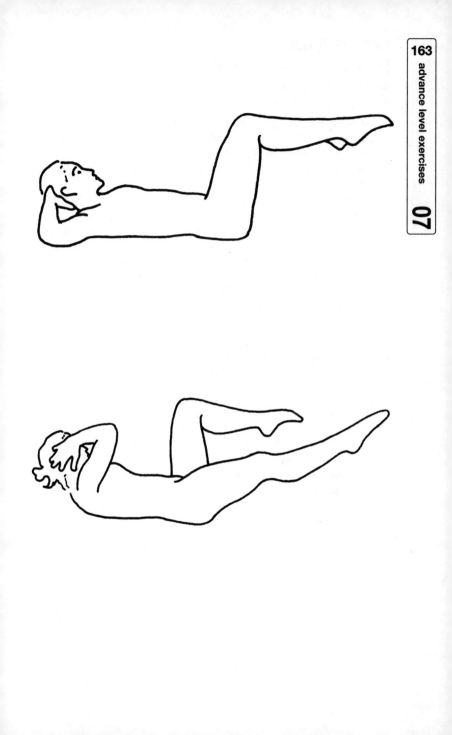

Leg pull lifted

Prelim exercises: Shoulder bridge, Plank with leg lifted

Benefits: Strengthens the triceps, the shoulders and all the muscles down the back to the ankles.

a Sit with your legs out straight in front of you. Place your hands on the mat, shoulder-width apart and just behind your hips, with your fingers facing towards your feet. Draw yourself up in the waist and push on your hands to lift your buttocks and the backs of your legs up off the mat. You are aiming to form a straight downward slope from your shoulders to your ankles.

b From your lifted position, breathe in as you lift your right leg straight up towards the ceiling. Breathe out as you lower your leg back down to the mat. Repeat this ten times with each leg before you lower yourself back down to the mat. From your sitting upright position take five controlled breaths and then repeat the exercise twice more.

Focus: Once you are in your lifted slope position you must keep your pelvis and spine fixed. You are using your core strength to maintain a fixed pelvis while lifting your legs.

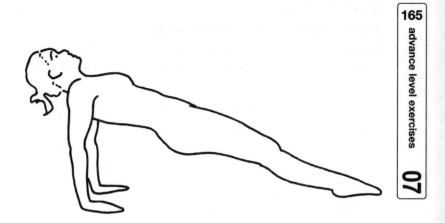

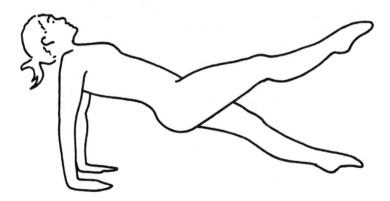

Teasing roll up

Prelim exercises: Full roll up, Leg pull balance

Benefits: Strengthens the abdominal muscles and the thighs. Improves control and balance while supporting and stretching the spine.

a Lie on your back with your legs out straight and your pelvis in the neutral position. Draw up your abdominal muscles and lift your legs to a 45-degree angle.

b Round the small of your back into the mat and breathe out as you begin rolling your body away from the mat and up towards your lifted legs. Keeping your abdominal muscles drawn up, sit up as high as you can without losing your balance.

c Breathe in as you lower your legs back down to the mat, and breathe out as you reach forward to stretch your spine.

d Breathe in as you lift yourself back into the sitting position with your legs lifted at a 45-degree angle, and breathe out as you roll your back slowly into the mat. When your arms are back down by your sides and your legs are still lifted take a breath in, and breathe out as you start to lift again.

Repeat the exercise 12 times.

Focus: Keep your abdominal muscles drawn up and control the movement from your waist. Obviously you should keep breathing, and in time your breathing pattern will become easier.

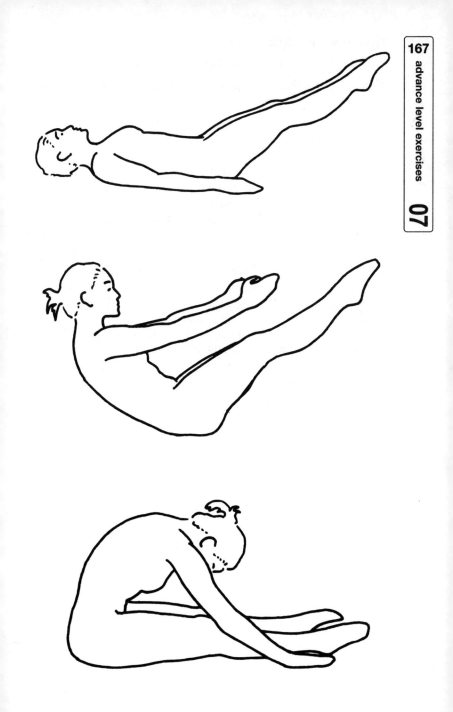

Open leg rocker

Prelim exercises: Roll up, Half-splits, The seal

Benefits: Strengthens the abdominal muscles, massages the back and improves balance.

a   Sit upright with your toes together and your knees bent and out to your sides. Place your hands on your shins and rest your elbows on your thighs.

b   Straighten your legs out into a V shape and hold your arms out straight. Draw up and tilt your pelvis towards you to create a C shape in your back. Breathe in as you tuck in your chin and begin to roll your back into the mat.

c   Keeping the C shape in your back, roll back as far as your shoulders, and breathe out as you roll back to your upright V position. Repeat this ten times, then take a 30-second rest before doing it again.

d   The higher you place your hands on your legs, the harder you have to work to control this exercise. If you are struggling, then move your hands down your legs to rest on your thighs. If you need a stronger challenge, hold your big toes while pointing your feet.

Focus: Keep the C shape in your back as you are rolling by using your abdominal muscles to keep control. Your hands are placed on your legs for support; you should not need to pull on them to control your roll.

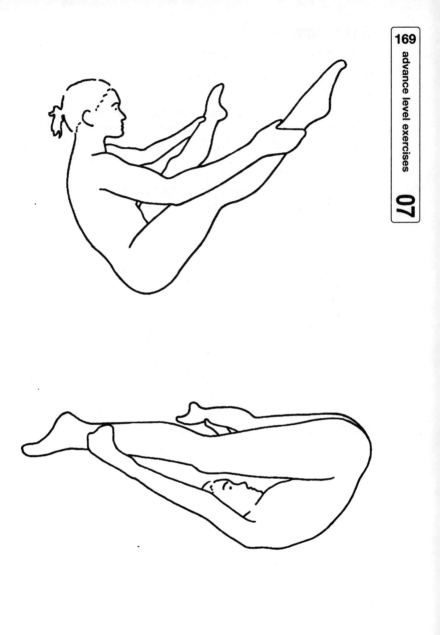

Arrow with triple kick

Prelim exercise: Swimming (lifted)

Benefits: Strengthens the back and legs; opens the chest and shoulders.

a Lie face down on your front with your head lifted an inch up from the mat, and place your hands on your lower back, palms up. Draw up and pull your navel away from the mat. Bend both knees and tap your heels on your bottom three times as you breathe out.

b Breathe in as you straighten and lift your legs as high as they will go while you are still resting on the tops of your thighs. At the same time lift your chest as you slide your shoulder blades down your back and open out your arms, palms facing away from your body.

c Think of yourself as an arrow in this more lifted position. Your chin stays down, and from your lower back to your neck there are no creases in your skin as you lengthen your body. Breathe out as you place your hands on your lower back and begin tapping your heels on your bottom. Repeat the movement 12 times, take a 30-second rest and do it again.

Focus: The abdominal muscles will be working hard at all stages of this exercise to stop your belly pushing out into the mat. Your upper back will be slightly extended, but the natural arch in your lower back should remain fixed. The erector spinae muscles in your back are working overtime to keep you lifted.

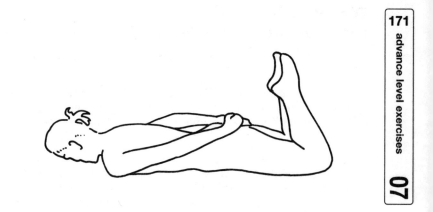

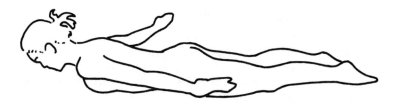

The saw

Prelim exercises: Open a book, Half-splits

Benefits: Rotates the spine; stretches the sides and the backs of the legs.

a Sit upright as if someone was pulling on the top of your head. Spread your legs wide and lift your arms up parallel with the floor, and with your hands out to the side just in front of your shoulders.

b Draw yourself up and breathe in as you rotate your body to the left. Breathe out as you reach out with your right arm towards your left shin. Take the stretch to a comfortable position, then breathe in as you gently release it, and breathe out as you reach forward towards your leg again twice more. Imagine that you are sawing your left leg with your right forearm for three movements.

c After your third sawing movement, breathe in and return to your upright rotated position. Breathe out as you come back to sitting upright, and repeat the exercise by rotating to the left and using your left arm to saw at your right leg. Complete five movements on each side.

Focus: Breathing in as you rotate your body helps you to lengthen and lift your spine as you twist. Keep your breathing slow on the sawing part of the exercise; there is no bouncing in the movement as you stretch yourself forward. As always, your abdominal muscles should remain drawn up as your arm reaches over to your leg, rather than collapsing your body to get closer.

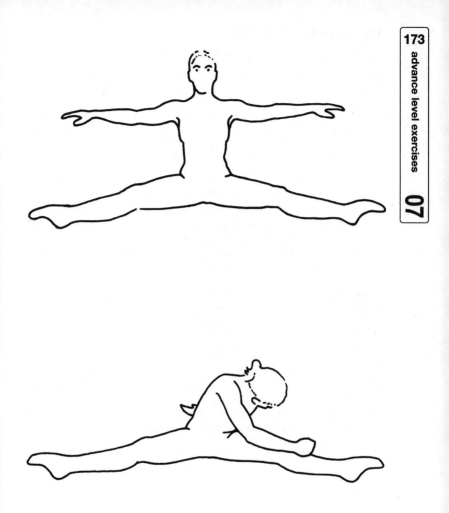

Double leg extension

Prelim exercises: Criss cross, Scissors

Benefits: Strengthens the front of the body, including the abdominal muscles and the lower back.

a Lie on your back with your knees bent and hip-width apart, and rest your head on the floor with the back of your neck lengthened. Draw up and fix your neutral pelvis position. Breathe in as you lift your legs, keeping them both bent, and rest your hands on your knees.

b Breathe out as you lift your head a couple of inches and straighten your legs while taking your arms up over your head; your rib cage must stay down, and the natural curve in your back stays completely fixed. Breathe in as you return to the bent leg position. Repeat this movement 12 times, and then hug your knees into your chest for 30 seconds before setting yourself back in your neutral position and repeating the whole exercise twice more.

c This is a very strong exercise; to increase the intensity drop your heels to within an inch of the floor and draw five very small circles in the air with your legs. Breathe in and out for five breaths before returning back to your bent knee position.

Focus: Lengthen your legs and arms away from your body as if someone is pulling at either end. I should be able to rest a cup of boiling water on your navel without fear of spilling a drop as you keep your waist area completely fixed.

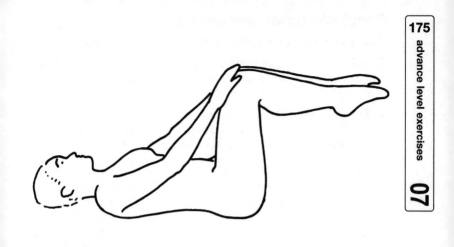

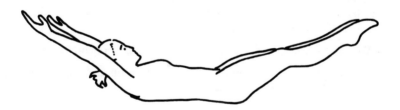

Chest and downward stretch

Prelim exercises: Hip hinge, Stomach and thigh stretch

Benefits: Stretches the front of the body, opening out the neck and chest, while the downward stretch works the back of the body from the ankles to the arms.

a Kneel on the mat with your knees a little wider than hip-width apart and the soles of your feet facing up to the ceiling. Draw up to support your back, and then gently reach back to place your left hand on your left foot. Keep your hips facing the front. With the weight on your left hand, slowly reach back to place your right hand on the sole of your right foot. Lower your head back, and hold this position for five slow breaths. To increase the stretch, push your hips forward while still keeping yourself drawn up. To come out of this position, bring your head forward and bend your knees to bring your bottom down.

b From a kneeling position with your hands on the floor, your knees under your hips and your toes tucked under your feet, draw up, push your heels to the mat, and lift your bottom up towards the ceiling. Your aim is to create a V shape with your body as you stretch the backs of your legs and your back. To increase the intensity of the stretch, walk your feet a little way back to bring your heels off the mat. Hold this for five slow breaths in and out.

After performing both exercises, repeat them once more.

Focus: Keep your abdominal muscles drawn up and enjoy your slow breathing in each posture.

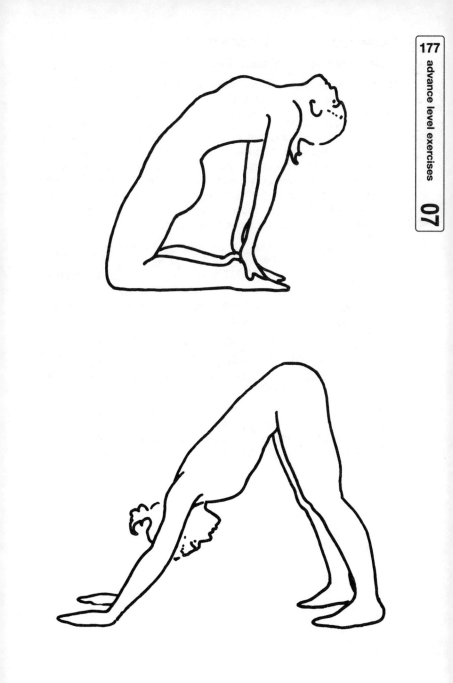

Table top

Prelim exercise: Hip hinge

Benefits: Strengthens and stretches the back and the legs to improve control and balance.

a Stand upright with your pelvis in the neutral position and your arms straight down by your sides. Draw yourself up and slowly bend forward so that you are hinging from your hip joints and not rounding your spine. As you hinge yourself forward, take your arms up above your head so that they are in line with your body. Your aim is to have your back level and parallel to the floor. Keep the back of your neck lengthened and do not let your head drop.

b Keeping the body fixed, lift up your right leg to bring it into line with the rest of your body. Except for the natural curves in your body, your back should be flat, resembling the top of a table. Take five slow breaths before controlling the lowering of your leg, and then return your body to an upright position. Repeat these moves on both sides twice.

c If you feel the need to intensify the balance of this exercise then lift up onto the ball of your foot while holding the tabletop position. Ensure that you do not let your ankle drop in or out while you are lifting.

Focus: Having strong abdominal muscles gives you increased control while balancing. Trying to focus on something fixed to the floor will also help you to control this movement, but do not let your head drop.

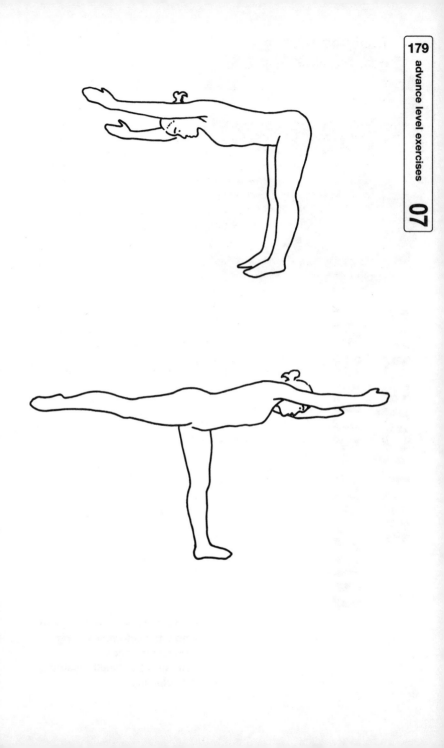

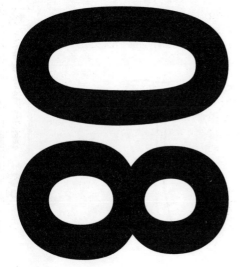

08

warm-down
stretches

In this chapter you will learn:
- how to perform warming down stretches
- about other health related disciplines.

Use this set of stretches after you have finished your exercise routine. Like the warm-up exercises, these movements have a set sequence. Many people who practise Eastern health techniques will know these stretches as the Makko-Ho exercises; don't worry if you do not. As with all stretches, take them to a point where you feel a gentle stretch and can still breathe comfortably. Fighting against your body to stretch will only make your body tense up in another area and restrict your breathing. If need be, spend a little more time exercising the areas of your body that feel tight, and allow yourself to sink further into the stretches. There is no rush!

The names for these stretches relate to the body's meridian channels in Chinese medicine. Whether you are interested in that or not, they are great stretches that work the whole body and leave you feeling lengthened and balanced.

Lung and large intestine

Stand with your feet shoulder-width apart and your knees slightly bent. Link your thumbs behind your back, and bend your stomach onto your thighs as you bring your arms up and over towards your head. Breathe slowly in and out for five breaths, and then drop your arms down onto your back before returning to your upright position. Then link your thumbs around the other way and repeat this movement.

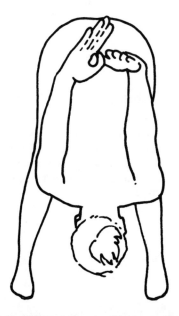

Stomach and spleen

Kneel down with your feet under your bottom. With your hands behind you, slowly lower your back closer to the mat. You are aiming to feel a comfortable stretch along the fronts of your thighs and your stomach. If you are quite flexible, you may get your back all the way down to the mat. Make sure there is no pain in your lower back, and hold this position for five breaths before coming out of the stretch.

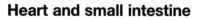

Heart and small intestine

Sit with your legs crossed, and your knees wide out to your sides. Place the heel of your right palm on your left knee and the heel of your left palm on your right knee. Keeping your knees spread out, gently pull on your knees until you feel a gentle stretch across your shoulders, then lower your head and hold this position for five breaths.

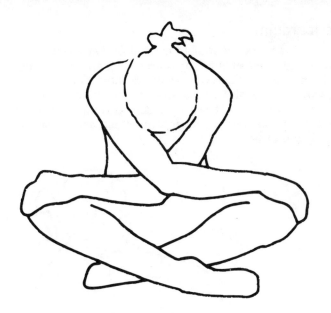

Bladder and kidney

Sit on the floor with the soles of your feet touching and your knees relaxed out to the sides. Gently pull on your ankles as you lean your chest down towards the floor, rounding your shoulders. Hold this position for five breaths.

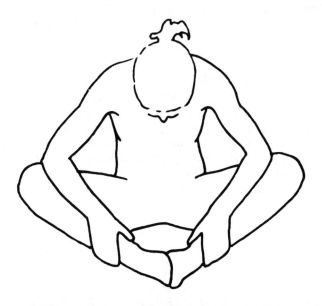

Pericardium

Sit with your legs out straight in front of you. Bend your arms so that the palms of your hands are facing away from you, but with the middle fingers touching. Breathe out as you bend forwards at the hips and push your hands away from you, towards your feet. Without bouncing, gently push your hands away from you every time you breathe out, and repeat this for five slow breaths.

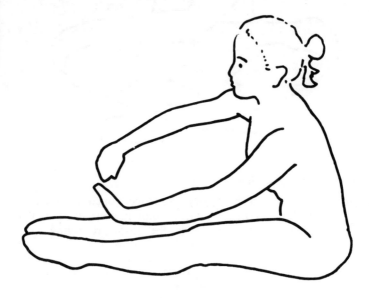

Liver and gall bladder

Sit upright on the floor with your legs wide apart. Bring your left foot into your groin and turn your waist, so that your nose and navel are pointing at your left knee. Gently lower your right ear towards your right knee and take your arms over to increase the stretch. Hold the position for five breaths before changing over to exercise the other side.

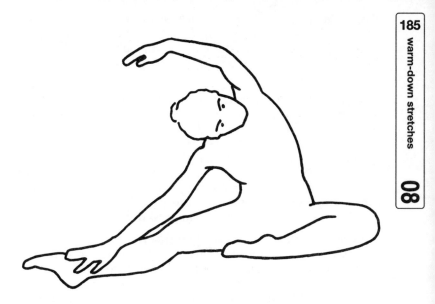

Various health related disciplines

When looking at improving your health through exercise the aim is to exercise in a way that is relative to your body, so that your body will be better suited to everyday life. There is a wide range of exercise techniques available, from the ancient breathing techniques of Yoga, the passive stretching of dance movements, and the body mechanics of weight training to bouncing on a physiotherapy ball. Some of the better-known practices are the Alexander Technique, Yoga and Tai Chi. These health related practices look at the body as a whole rather than as just a structure, and they have a proven record in improving health.

With the Alexander Technique, you relearn to move your body in the way it was designed to move. The practice accepts the fact that the stresses and strains of life play a role in affecting the shape and possible misalignment of the body. Exercises and new ways of thinking help to unlearn conditioned bad habits. Realizing you have a choice about how to react physically and emotionally gives you a more positive outlook on life.

The technique can be traced back to the founder, Frederick Matthis Alexander, who himself was inspired by his own ailments to find a more efficient way of holding and using his body. He was born in 1869 and his technique has been practised over the last 100 years.

Yoga is another form of exercise that takes into account more than just the physical aspects of our bodies. It aims to bring unity and balance to our body and mind through focused breathing, stretching techniques and internal exercises. It has its own philosophy and requires a high level of dedication to reach the higher levels of practice. However, the beginner can still benefit from it, as there are many challenging aspects to Yoga which give suitability for all. Its history can be traced back over 2,500 years through ancient Indian Sanskrit texts.

Tai Chi is another health related art that is suitable for all ages and levels. Its beautiful flowing movements provide an awareness of how you should hold your body. It teaches focusing the mind, toning the muscles and keeping the body supple with the least amount of tension in the joints. Its gentle yet energetic postures help build strength into everyday movements. Like Yoga it has a long history and its own philosophy relating to the balancing effects of Yin and Yang. During the Chinese Cultural Revolution in the 1970s, the government recommended that all people over a certain age should take up the practice of Tai Chi, and many senior citizens can still be seen practising this ancient art form.

As with Pilates, each one of these techniques can complement the others. Obviously there is not enough time to become proficient at all of these practices in one go; it makes sense to focus your energies on perfecting one technique before rushing into the next.

Pilates offers a simple way of improving your body's health and shape. It does require patience and dedication, but so does anything worthwhile. All of these health practices require you to get some hands-on experience from an experienced teacher. A book can set you on the right path, but a teacher can provide you with a progressive understanding of the technique. Many teachers of Pilates are closely associated with physiotherapy and osteopathy clinics, and as new information is uncovered through research, improved exercises are created. This makes Pilates a living therapy.

Good health

Our ability to carry out our daily tasks with vigour and a positive attitude and still have energy left over at the end of the day for extra activities is for most of us a sign of good health. If we lack this extra energy and our bodies always ache, or if we cannot shrug off a simple cold, we would rightly consider ourselves to be unhealthy. When we look at others we can quickly gauge in our own minds whether they look healthy or not. The evidence on which we draw might be the sparkle in their eyes, the fresh bloom in their cheeks, the size of their stomach or their general get-up-and-go attitude. The ability to complete a ten-mile run is not necessarily a sign of good health; nor would we associate good health with someone who goes to the gym each day but is always tired and complains of a bad back. These people could be overdoing it and actually depleting their energy levels rather than building them up.

Think of the health of your body as a bank account. We all start off with varying levels of cash, some with more than others. With a balanced level of exercise, whether it is naturally gained through physical exercise at work, going for long walks or more focused on specific exercising routines, we are maintaining or depositing extra savings in our health bank account. As we get older we naturally use up our reserves, and if we are ill or injured we put more of a strain on our health bank accounts; but if you are continually spending without replenishing your account through resting, good diet and sensible exercise, then something is going to give. This could be a simple injury or illness that forces you either to rest or to take up a form of rehabilitating exercise. On the other hand it could be a life-threatening illness that will totally change your life. My aim is not to frighten anyone, but time spent working on improving your health is time well spent. I appreciate that having a nice big house, a shiny new car or even a big swimming pool are pleasurable goals, but these goals are nothing compared with your health. Imagine your last words on your deathbed as being, 'I wish I'd had a bigger house.' I don't think so! It is more likely that you would say 'I wish I'd had more energy to play with my grandchildren' or 'I would have liked to walk on the Great Wall of China'. Whatever your aspirations or situation in life, with improved health your body will be better equipped to enjoy them.

The realistic bonus for spending some time improving your fitness is that you feel good and you are on a natural energetic high. This improves your mental attitude and stamina, which in turn could probably make you better at your job. Indeed it may be that without even trying too hard you could end up with the swimming pool. If so, give me a ring and I will bring my swimming trunks!

Just as physical well being has a positive effect on our mental state, so feeling good mentally can also affect the way we feel physically. A bad day at work, when our colleagues are miserable and complaining or even targeting us about our failure to achieve something, can leave us feeling tired and drained at the end of the day. Dealing with a variety of different and difficult emotions that can be thrown at your body throughout the day can be very tiring, but remember that you have a choice about how to react to what others are doing to you. Our moods and the way we feel are under our control. When we get out of our beds in the morning and look at ourselves in the mirror we have the choice to say something positive to ourselves that will help our mental attitude throughout the day. Being healthy and fit gives us a more balanced outlook on how to deal with life's sometimes difficult decisions and situations.

What we eat and drink plays a big part in our health, too, and the phrase 'you are what you eat' is well founded. Unfortunately one person's medicine can be another person's poison and we are all different in respect of the foodstuffs that are most suitable for our bodies. Moderation is definitely the key. If you do not want to be fat, and chips and cream cakes make you fat, then you are going to have to eat less. If mixing proteins and carbohydrates makes you feel bloated and lethargic, then you have the choice not to mix them. Through information, or trial and error, we find out which foodstuffs agree with our digestive system and which ones are less suitable. The more you start to appreciate and feel what is better for you, the less time you will want to spend consuming unsuitable foodstuffs. The more you realize that regular balanced exercise will help you to maintain a healthier outlook on life, the easier it will be to spend time getting and staying fit.

The fact that you are reading this page shows that you care about your health and that you are already making, or are about to make, an effort to look after yourself. Do not worry about your age or state of fitness; it is never too late. There is one lady in my class who is 90 years old and she finds that the classes leave her feeling very balanced. Pilates will not meet all your fitness needs but it will give your body a solid foundation of strength and support that can stand alone or be added to any other fitness programme. As you become more in tune with your body's movements it will encourage you to maintain and improve your health.

As a human being your potential for achievement is almost limitless; it makes sense, therefore, to exercise both your body and your mind. Your body is the vehicle in which you travel through life and your brain controls the directions in which you go. You owe it to yourself to look after them both.

Good luck and good health.

These days most gyms offer Pilates classes at a variety of levels. In large classes don't be shy. Stand at the front and let the teacher know of any previous experience or problems. If, however, you are new to exercise, returning after a long interval, or suffering from a minor injury, it would be preferable to look for a small, specialized class or personal tuition. Your local physiotherapist or physiotherapy clinic should be able to recommend a suitable class or instructor. For example, I work at the Manor Clinic, Sevenoaks, Kent.

A search of the term 'Pilates' on the Internet will reveal a host of websites, institutions, classes and publications. There are numerous books about Pilates, but those with an interest in history may prefer to go directly to *The Complete Writings of Joseph H Pilates*, see, for example the collection edited by Gallagher and Kryzanowska, published by Bainbridge Books in 2000.

Related books in the *Teach Yourself* series include *Alexander Technique*, *Anatomy and Physiology*, *Tai Chi* and *Yoga*. For those seeking a further understanding of the body and how it works see the *Anatomy of Movement* and *Anatomy of Movement Exercises* volumes published by Eastland Press. Paul Blakey, *The Muscle Book*, published by Bibliotek books, provides a brief but clear introduction to the subject while Justin Howse and Shirley Hancock, *Dance Technique and Injury Prevention*, published by A & C Black, is a key specialist work.

index

| teach yourself | **yoga**
mary stewart |

- Are you interested in the origins and history of yoga?
- Do you want to find out if yoga might be right for you?
- Would you like to make it part of your everyday life?

Yoga explains both the theory and practice of yoga. With clear, step-by-step illustrations it explains yoga breathing and meditation and shows you how to perform the poses, to promote flexibility and strength and relieve the stress of everyday living. Find out how this ancient system of meditation and exercise can transform your life!

Mary Stewart has been teaching yoga for over 30 years and is the author of five books on the subject.

| teach yourself | **alexander technique** |
| | richard craze |

- Would you like to learn a new approach to health?
- Are you looking for a therapy to help back problems?
- Do you want to benefit from this effective method of re-educating the body?

Alexander Technique is a complete, no-nonsense reference guide to an increasingly popular alternative therapy in which realignment of the spine and body provides stress relief and an enhanced sense of well-being. This book explores the history of the technique and how it was developed, and includes practical exercises to maximize your understanding.

Richard Craze is a freelance writer specializing in books on alternative health, new age, religion and other esoteric subjects.

teach
yourself

reflexology
chris stormer

- Are you new to reflexology?
- Would you like to learn a different approach to good health?
- Do you want to relieve stress?

Reflexology will help you to discover this ancient and gentle form of healing, which uses reflex points on the feet to stimulate the body's natural ability to heal itself. The step-by-step instructions and many illustrations give even the complete beginner the information and confidence to get started right away.

Chris Stormer is an acknowledged authority on reflexology. She is the founder of the Reflexology Academy of Southern Africa and holds workshops and lectures worldwide.

| teach yourself | # human anatomy & physiology
david le vay |

- Do you need to know basic anatomy for a course or profession?
- Are you interested in how the body works?
- Do you want to understand more about scientific innovation?

Human Anatomy and Physiology is a comprehensive introduction to the structure and function of the human body. Extensively illustrated, the book also covers modern methods of investigation, relevant aspects of modern genetics, sports injuries, environmental and evolutionary considerations and the physiological aspects of AIDS.

David le Vay MS, FRCS was a consultant surgeon for many years and a well-known medical author and editor.

teach
yourself

massage
denise whichello brown

- Do you want to understand the principles of massage?
- Would you like your life to benefit from this popular technique?
- Do you need a simple introduction in preparation for a course of study?

Massage gives a complete guide to this ancient and popular technique. Learn how to apply the basic principles to relieve stress, to treat sports injuries or to develop your personal relationships. The text is extensively illustrated with clear, fully labelled diagrams.

Denise Whichello Brown is a highly acclaimed practitioner, lecturer and author of international repute, with over 20 years' experience in complementary medicine.

tai chi
robert parry

- Do you want to understand the basic principles of Tai Chi?
- Would you like step-by-step instructions for the movements?
- Are you looking for an antidote to a stressful lifestyle?

Tai Chi explores the background and philosophy of Tai Chi and gives clear instructions for learning the 'short yang form', suitable for all ages and all levels of fitness. Introduce Tai Chi into your everyday life and reap the benefits of this centuries-old system of exercise from China.

Robert Parry is a practitioner of oriental medicine and has been active in the study of Eastern systems of exercise and philosophy for over 30 years